LAURENCE E. STEMPEL

D1204614

LAURENCE E. STEMPEL

Atlas of Obstetric technic

Atlas of
Obstetric technic

J. Robert Willson, M.D., M.S.

Professor of Obstetrics and Gynecology, The University of Michigan Medical School; Chairman of the Department of Obstetrics and Gynecology, University of Michigan Medical Center, Ann Arbor, Michigan

Second edition

With 58 plates including 375 illustrations by Daisy Stilwell

The C. V. Mosby Company

Saint Louis   1969

Second edition

Copyright © 1969 by The C. V. Mosby Company

All rights reserved. No part of this book may be reproduced in any manner without written permission of the publisher.

Previous edition copyrighted 1961

Printed in the United States of America

Standard Book Number 8016-5591-9

Library of Congress Catalog Card Number 70-95649

Distributed in Great Britain by Henry Kimpton, London

Preface

An author must of necessity justify his decision to revise a textbook of operative technic since the technical details of operative procedures vary little from year to year. If the decision to prepare a new edition of the *Atlas of Obstetric Technic* had been based only upon the need to alter the procedures described in the first edition or to add new operations, a revision would have been unnecessary. As stated in the preface to the first edition, "I have attempted to include enough text to make this book more than a collection of drawings of operations." It is the text, therefore, rather than the illustrations that has been changed. The section concerning the use of oxytocin for the induction of labor and for stimulation of dysfunctional labor has been rewritten, as has that on the management of the third stage of labor. Newer methods of placental localization are described. The use of the measurement of urinary estriol excretion and of the examination of amniotic fluid in an attempt to assess the status of the fetus in utero is described in appropriate places. A number of changes in recommendations for managing labor complicated by abnormal fetal positions have been made. The portion devoted to obstetric analgesia and anesthesia has been expanded. The new illustrations included in this area were prepared by Mr. Grant Lashbrook of the Medical and Biological Illustration Unit of the University of Michigan.

The concept that the book serve principally as a reference for residents and practicing physicians with a background in obstetrics has been retained. Although the book should be of greatest value to those who are actively practicing obstetrics, it can also be used to advantage by medical students. The step-by-step illustration of normal delivery and of the maneuvers designed to solve the various abnormalities that may complicate labor should provide the student with a means of understanding the reasons for and the effects of such complications and the ways in which they can be solved. I trust that all these physicians will find the book helpful to them and ultimately to their patients.

J. Robert Willson

v

Contents

Atlas of Obstetric technic

Chapter 1

The professional staff; labor and delivery room facilities

The increased safety with which women can have babies is in part a result of the expansion of hospital obstetric facilities and a concurrent decrease in home delivery. Naturally the application of the advances in general medical knowledge, the availability of blood transfusion, the development of antimicrobial substances, and improved anesthetic and surgical technics have also played a part in reducing maternal and infant mortality. Of at least equal importance is the fact that general practitioners have been better prepared in medical school and during their internships to manage normal labor and delivery and to recognize complications, and more trained and competent specialists are available for consultation when an abnormality does arise.

However, no matter how dedicated and skillful a physician may be, he is helpless when a complication arises unless the necessary facilities for its treatment are readily available for immediate use. One of the major responsibilities of the chief of an obstetric service and his staff is to determine what physical facilities, instruments, medications, and personnel are necessary for the care of normal pregnant women and those with complications, and to check periodically to make certain that they are available. If a department is inadequately equipped and consequently not prepared to render the best possible treatment, it usually is because the physicians have done nothing to correct obvious deficiencies. This often is a result of the fact that the department has not been well organized and, as a consequence, no single individual has authority either to establish policy or to act as the liaison agent between the staff members and the administrator.

1

STAFF ORGANIZATION

The professional staff may consist entirely of specialists, entirely of family physicians, or a combination of both. However, regardless of distribution, one individual should be appointed as the executive officer. Whenever possible, he should be an experienced, qualified specialist who is familiar with obstetric problems and who can develop and supervise nurse, intern, and resident training programs, establish policy, enforce departmental rules, and serve as professional consultant and as arbitrator whenever a difference of opinion concerning policy or patient management arises. It is important that he be interested in organizing and developing the department and willing to allocate a sufficient amount of time to the job. A chief should not be appointed because he is the most popular member of the staff or has the largest practice, or because it is his turn to serve. He should be appointed for a term of at least three years and should be eligible for reappointment if he has discharged his responsibilities ably and wishes to continue.

PROFESSIONAL PRIVILEGES AND CONSULTATION

Blanket privileges cannot logically be given simply because an individual is or claims to be a specialist nor be withheld because he has not had special training, because general practitioners may be more able and conscientious obstetricians than are some of those who have had formal obstetric and gynecologic training. The chief of the service, with the help of a committee of unbiased and competent obstetricians, should determine what each individual department member is permitted to do. Privileges may be expanded or reduced depending upon the activities of the individual as reviewed from time to time.

The conditions for which consultation is required or recommended should be clearly established for each individual and, as with operative privileges, are determined upon the basis of proved ability rather than rank. The most capable senior staff members are designated as consultants, and the other staff members should be encouraged to consult with them whenever a problem is anticipated or encountered. The free use of consultation can be encouraged if the consultant serves only as a consultant (offering advice, assisting in the delivery, or performing difficult operative procedures himself when necessary) and does not take over the entire care of the patient, finally appropriating her completely. If the latter situation occurs regularly, physicians will understandably be loath to ask for help.

In general there should be no fee for single consultations within the department; this is particularly true when consultation is mandatory. If the consultant must visit the patient several times, supervise unusual examinations or treatment, or actually deliver her, a fee is justifiable.

For the *specialist of proved ability*, consultation is desirable whenever a patient has a major complication. For *nonspecialists*, consultation should be required before any cesarean section, before induction of labor, for patients who make unsatisfactory progress during twelve hours of either active or dysfunctional labor, in cases of malpresentation, hemorrhage, toxemia, major medical complications, and serious lacerations, and before performing operative delivery of any type.

LABOR AND DELIVERY ROOMS—PHYSICAL FACILITIES

The labor and the delivery rooms should be separated from the rest of the hospital, and the nursing staff should have no responsibilities in other areas.

Admitting room. An examining room in which patients who are being considered for admission to the labor-delivery area can be seen is desirable. Such a facility permits the screening of patients before they actually are placed in a labor room, thereby preventing the admission of women with infections, those who do not need to enter the hospital, and those who are best admitted to another patient care area. Such a room is best placed near the labor area and should be equipped with an examining table, sterile gloves and instruments, syringes, test tubes, etc. for obtaining blood, catheter trays, an accurate scale, a shower, and a toilet. The entire evaluation of the patient can be performed in the admitting room. If such a facility is not available, the patient can be seen and examined in the labor room in which she will remain until she is ready for delivery.

A small laboratory equipped for blood counts and urine examination is desirable unless reports can be obtained promptly at any hour from the hospital's general laboratory.

Prelabor rooms. Patients with ruptured membranes, those in early or preliminary labor, and those who may be in false labor are usually more comfortable in a facility separate from the labor and delivery rooms. When possible, this should be near the delivery area for ease in following the patient's progress. When this cannot be arranged, such patients may be sent to the obstetric floor until more active treatment becomes necessary.

Labor rooms. The suggested ratio of one labor bed for each 250 deliveries a year may be inadequate if the former must be used for women in questionable or preliminary labor or as recovery beds. Single labor rooms are preferable to multiple bed units, even though the beds are screened or are in cubicles, and they should be soundproofed and well ventilated or air conditioned. The doors should be wide enough to permit the labor bed to be wheeled in and out without difficulty. Suction equipment and a source of oxygen should be readily available. Each room should contain a bed with side rails, a straight chair and a more comfortable chair, a sphygmomanometer, a stethoscope, a fetoscope, a supply of gloves, lubricant, and a writing surface. Toilet facilities and wash basins must be in the immediate vicinity, and a call system is essential. There should be a utility room in the area for preparation and storage of equipment and linen.

Medications, except those used during and immediately after delivery, should be stored and prepared in the labor room area.

Two bottles of Rh-negative type O blood should be stored in the refrigerator ready for immediate administration in the event of an overwhelming hemorrhage. The blood should be replaced as soon as it has been used; if it is not needed, fresh blood should be substituted every three or four days. Five percent saline solution, 20% dextrose in water, and some sort of plasma expander, as well as the necessary equipment for their intravenous administration, should be provided. A sterile cut-down set should be readily available. A constant supply of fibrinogen is essential.

Delivery rooms. Delivery rooms are used for no other purpose and are equipped like an operating room. Each should contain a suitable delivery table, stools for the anesthetist and the obstetrician, a completely equipped anesthetic machine, and all the instruments that may be necessary for normal or operative delivery, for postdelivery examination of the birth canal, and for the repair of lacerations. A heated crib should be adjacent to a suction apparatus and a supply of oxygen, and the necessary equipment for tracheal intubation and resuscitation of the infant must be at hand. Materials for identification of the infant are also important. Equipment and solution for intravenous therapy must be available.

Delivery room medications include oxytocics (such as methylergonovine [Methergine], ergonovine [Ergotrate], and oxytocin), epinephrine (Adrenalin), ephedrine, phenylephrine (Neo-Synephrine), methoxamine hydrochloride (Vasoxyl), and nalorphine (Nalline). If others are needed, they can be obtained from the supply in the labor room.

One delivery room should be equipped with an operating table and instruments for the performance of emergency cesarean section. This room can also be used for vaginal deliveries.

Women with definite infections must be isolated from the rest of the labor patients. This can be accomplished by conducting the entire labor and delivery in a labor room or a delivery room. The rooms must be cleaned before other patients are admitted to them.

The linen and instruments used in the labor and delivery rooms should be kept separate from those used in the rest of the hospital. They are most easily processed and stored in workrooms, sterilizing rooms, and storage rooms in the delivery room area.

Recovery rooms. A recovery area in which the patient can be kept under constant observation until she has reacted and seems to be progressing normally provides an additional safety factor. One nurse can check several patients, recording pulse rate and blood pressure, palpating the fundus, and watching for abnormal bleeding. The normal patients usually are kept in the area for an hour or so before being taken to their rooms, and patients with complications are usually kept until they no longer need continual care and can be moved safely. Labor rooms can be used as recovery rooms if there are enough of them.

Chapter 2

Normal labor and delivery

ADMISSION

The patient who enters the hospital for delivery is conducted to an admitting area where she is questioned and examined to determine whether she actually is in active labor and, if so, how far it has advanced. These decisions are best made by a physician, who should see the patient promptly after she reaches the admitting room. If he finds that labor is in progress and that there are no obvious abnormalities, he performs a complete physical examination, determines the hemoglobin concentration or the hematocrit level, and tests the urine for protein and sugar. It is not necessary to shave the pubis, but the vulvar and perineal hair should usually be removed. If the rectum is filled with fecal material, an enema or a suppository may be administered. Neither is necessary if the presenting part has descended deeply into the pelvis or if the cervix is well dilated and labor is advancing rapidly. An enema is contraindicated if there is unexplained vaginal bleeding. Patients may use the toilet during early labor. However, primigravidas who are well along in the first stage and most multiparas whose contractions are recurring frequently should use a bedpan.

CARE DURING LABOR

After the patient has been prepared, she is transferred to a labor room, where she will remain until she is ready for delivery. Many women are more comfortable in a chair than in a bed during early labor. However, as the contractions become stronger, they usually prefer to lie down. Any patient who has had medication should be confined to a bed with protective side rails to prevent her from falling out if she is disoriented or unusually active. No patient who has been sedated should be left alone.

The gastric emptying time is prolonged in women in labor, particularly those to whom sedatives have been given. Food and fluid ingested during labor will remain in the stomach and may be regurgitated and aspirated when an anesthetic is administered for delivery. This complication can be

5

avoided by prohibiting patients from taking any type of food or fluid orally until they have been delivered. Medications are administered hypodermically, and fluids that are necessary to prevent dehydration during prolonged labors or in unusually hot weather are given intravenously.

Each patient and her infant in the labor area must be constantly attended by a physician or a trained and experienced labor nurse, because an alert observer can often detect complications at their onset or even anticipate them before they develop. The blood pressure should be taken and recorded and the fetal heart rate counted at least every half hour. If either is abnormal, more frequent observation is necessary.

PAIN RELIEF DURING LABOR

Some women, particularly those who have been trained in one of the psychoprophylactic methods, can go through an entire labor and even deliver the baby without any great discomfort, but for most the process is painful. The severity of the pain can almost always be reduced to a tolerable level without adding to the risk of either the mother or her infant and without eliminating consciousness in the former. Although a patient must never be forced to take sedative drugs, suitable methods for reducing discomfort should be made available to those who want them. There can be no routine method for relieving pain during labor, because the needs of patients vary, and that which may be quite adequate for one may be contraindicated for another. Each dosage of medication should be prescribed by a physician, who makes his decision as to which particular drug or combination of drugs to use and the amount to be administered on the basis of the duration of pregnancy, the stage of labor, the patient's reactions to labor, and the condition of the infant.

Systemic analgesia. The pain during the early part of the first stage of labor is relatively slight, but many patients are somewhat anxious and tense. During this period ataraxic preparations are more suitable than opiates. Promethazine hydrochloride (Phenergan), 50 to 100 mg., or another similar preparation will usually relax the patient between contractions and keep her reasonably comfortable until the pain becomes more severe. These preparations do not influence uterine activity and will not interfere with the normal progress of labor.

Most women become uncomfortable by the time the cervix has dilated 4 to 5 cm., and if labor is progressing normally and the mother requests medication, an analgesic drug can be administered at this stage. All drugs given to the mother cross the placenta and affect the infant; consequently, the dosage of the preparation used should be no more than the amount thought necessary to control discomfort. The physician's aim should be to reduce pain rather than to eliminate it completely. The patient who is properly sedated will be relaxed between contractions but will be able to cooperate with the attendants and respond logically.

Meperidine (Demerol) or *morphine* will control the pain adequately, and either may be administered to normal patients. The effectiveness of both is enhanced by the addition of an *ataraxic preparation.* For the first injection, 50 mg. Demerol or 6 to 8 mg. morphine sulfate and 50 mg. Phenergan will usually produce the desired reaction in the mother. If an ataraxic drug has already been used during the early stages of labor, it is well to eliminate it or at least reduce the dosage when the opiate is administered. If the patient had Phenergan more than six hours previously, an additional 50 mg. may be given with the first injection of Demerol; if Phenergan was given two to four hours previously, the second dose should be reduced to 25 mg.; if it was given less than two hours previously, the opiate alone may be given.

In most multiparas there is no need to use more than a single injection of medication during the entire labor; however, in primigravidas it may be necessary to reinforce the original amount after four to six hours. A second injection of 50 mg. Phenergan combined with 50 mg. Demerol or 6 to 8 mg. morphine sulfate usually will control the patient's discomfort until delivery is imminent.

It is unwise to give Demerol or morphine to patients who will probably deliver within an hour and a half or two hours, because the infant may be born while still somewhat depressed by the drug. Late in the first stage the patient may be given 60 mg. alphaprodine (Nisentil) intramuscularly if delivery is not anticipated within an hour. The action of this drug is much shorter than that of morphine or Demerol.

Gas analgesia. The discomfort toward the end of the first stage of labor can also be controlled by intermittent inhalations of *nitrous oxide* (75% to 80%) and *oxygen* (20% to 25%). The gas is administered by an anesthetist during each contraction. It is most effective if the patient begins to inhale the mixture as soon as a contraction can be palpated by an attendant rather than when she first becomes aware of discomfort.

Regional analgesia. The pain during labor can also be controlled with *caudal* or *epidural* anesthesia, which can be continued as the anesthetic for delivery. Caudal and epidural technics are particularly advantageous during premature labor and for women with heart disease, pulmonary disease, and diabetes because they control pain and relax the voluntary pelvic muscles without interfering either with uterine contractions or with oxygenation of the infant. Caudal or epidural anesthesia is more useful in primigravidas than in multiparas in whom short labors and easy deliveries can be anticipated. They should be administered only by trained individuals who can remain with the patients during the entire labor and reinforce the initial injections whenever the pain recurs.

Pain can also be relieved with *paracervical block*, in which the anesthetic agent is injected superficially in each vaginal fornix just lateral to the cervix. This technic is effective for both multiparas and primigravidas.

7

When the termination of the second stage of labor is imminent, the patient is moved from the labor area to the delivery room in which her infant will be born. In most instances, the move is accomplished most rapidly and safely by wheeling the patient in her bed rather than placing her on a stretcher, because, as sometimes happens, the head or the entire infant may be born while she is being moved from bed to litter or from litter to delivery table. If the number of such transfers can be kept to a minimum, the chance of the baby's being injured by falling is reduced.

ANESTHESIA

A few women, particularly those with relaxed or unusually elastic pelvic supporting structures, can be delivered with minimal anesthesia or none at all, but some form of pain relief usually is desirable for normal delivery and is essential for operative delivery. Since no single method is suitable for routine use, the obstetrician should have several anesthetic technics available from which he can select the one most appropriate for each patient.

Inhalation anesthesia. Some women demand inhalation anesthesia either because they are fearful of conduction methods or because they want to be unconscious during the birth of the baby. General anesthesia is quite satisfactory when it is properly administered; however, there are certain hazards that accompany its use. The most serious complication is *vomiting* and *aspiration,* as a result of which many mothers die each year. The incidence of aspiration can be reduced by forbidding the ingestion of food and fluids after uterine contractions begin. If a patient has eaten recently, a regional technic should be used or her stomach emptied before a general anesthetic is administered.

Prolonged deep inhalation anesthesia will *reduce the intensity of uterine contractions,* thus increasing both the need for operative delivery and the incidence of serious bleeding in the third stage of labor. The infant can also be depressed by prolonged anesthesia, with a *resultant delay in onset of respiration* following his delivery. With the exception of vomiting, these complications generally need not occur when general anesthesia is used for normal delivery.

Nitrous oxide–oxygen mixtures alone may provide enough pain relief for normal spontaneous delivery but are generally inadequate for the performance of episiotomy and forceps extraction unless the oxygen content is reduced to a dangerously low level. Deeper anesthesia can be obtained by adding *ether* or *trichloroethylene* to the mixture. The analgesic effect of nitrous oxide–oxygen is usually better if the gas has been administered intermittently during the second stage of labor than if it is started when the patient is in the process of expelling the infant.

Ether has a wide margin of safety as an obstetric anesthetic agent. However, when given alone, it is unpleasant for the patient and the induction time is prolonged. For the usual delivery it is used most effectively to reinforce the anesthetic effect of nitrous oxide–oxygen mixtures. Most deliveries can be successfully accomplished using this combination. An important use of ether is the provision of complete uterine relaxation for breech extraction or version. It is one of the few agents with which uterine activity can be abolished safely. The induction time is prolonged to fifteen to twenty minutes, and bleeding will be increased because of the inhibition of uterine contractions. The blood loss can be minimized if the anesthetic is stopped when the version is completed or the legs are brought down in a breech position; during the extraction the patient will usually recover to a point at which spontaneous uterine contractions will recur.

Trichloroethylene (Trilene) is an analgesic agent that can be used alone for rapid spontaneous delivery but generally is inadequate for operative extraction. It can be used effectively to reinforce the effect of nitrous oxide–oxygen if certain precautions are taken. It should never be given in a closed-circuit apparatus because it combines with soda lime to produce phosgene and dichloracetylene. For the same reason a closed-circuit machine should not be used to anesthetize a patient who has inhaled Trilene during labor. Trilene also may cause cardiac arrhythmia when given in too high a concentration. Although the nitrous oxide–oxygen–trichloroethylene combination is effective, it should be administered by an experienced anesthetist and with machines that have been converted for its use.

Cyclopropane has advantages and disadvantages as an obstetric anesthetic agent. It produces good uterine relaxation, and the induction is rapid and relatively pleasant and can be accomplished with a high concentration of oxygen. The ease and rapidity with which a patient can be induced, however, may be a disadvantage unless an experienced anesthetist is in charge. An anesthetic level far deeper than that necessary for the contemplated delivery will often result, and the infant may be depressed despite the high oxygen concentration; this is particularly true when the anesthetic time exceeds eight to ten minutes.

Conduction anesthesia. Conduction, or regional, anesthesia, when properly used, is generally safer than inhalation anesthesia for both the mother and her infant. It does not alter the uterine contraction pattern significantly and, unless the maternal blood pressure falls, does not interfere with oxygenation of the baby. The methods of conduction anesthesia that depend upon nerve root block (spinal, caudal, and epidural) are more hazardous than those which anesthetize the peripheral nerves (local infiltration and pudendal nerve block).

Nerve root block. Caudal and epidural anesthesia provide excellent pain relief and relaxation of the pelvic muscles without affecting the uterine contractions or fetal oxygenation. Since it takes some time to insert the needle or catheter properly and to obtain an effective anesthetic level, it is more satisfactory when used as an analgesic during labor and continued as an anesthetic for delivery than when administered only as a terminal anesthetic. Caudal and epidural technics are not satisfactory for general use because of the potential dangers (massive intrathecal injection and infection), because of the need for constant supervision by experienced individuals, and because many women do not need this much anesthesia. They are of particular value for women with heart disease, pulmonary disorders, and metabolic disorders such as diabetes, and during premature labor and delivery.

Saddle block, or *low spinal anesthesia,* provides excellent pain relief and pelvic muscle relaxation but is potentially the most dangerous of all the methods. Unless it is given with the greatest of care by experienced individuals to carefully selected patients, the mortality will be higher than with any other anesthetic. The principal cause of death is shock and respiratory paralysis from an ascending level of anesthesia, either because too much of the agent was administered or because of improper technic. It is most often used for the delivery of primigravidas. However, it provides excellent anesthesia and voluntary muscle relaxation for more difficult forceps rotation and extraction. Spinal anesthesia has little effect upon uterine muscle contraction; consequently, it is not suitable for version and extraction or for breech extraction except for the operative delivery of an infant in complete breech position when the feet lie in the vagina and can be reached without inserting the entire hand and forearm into the uterine cavity.

Intrathecal anesthesia is contraindicated in women who are bleeding profusely or who are in shock, those with moderately severe hypertension, those who have diseases of the central nervous system or spine, those with local infections near the proposed puncture site, those who claim sensitivity to local anesthetic agents, and particularly those who wish to be asleep or who fear spinal anesthesia.

I prefer the saddle block technic, using 3 to 5 mg. Pontocaine in 10% dextrose, which usually provides a level of anesthesia to about the tenth thoracic vertebra. The blood pressure, pulse rate, and fetal heart tones must be checked every minute for at least ten minutes, by which time a stable level has usually been obtained. A fall in blood pressure from vasodilation in the anesthetized area may reduce uterine blood flow and fetal oxygenation, which will be indicated by a decrease in fetal heart rate. If this does occur, it can usually be corrected by raising the mother's legs and administering oxygen.

Peripheral nerve block. Local block of the peripheral nerves can be used successfully to relieve the pain accompanying the delivery of most multiparas and many primigravidas. Women who are unusually fearful, those who react poorly to discomfort, and those who are unusually active are poor candidates for local anesthesia. The procedures are safe, simple, and effective, require a minimum of equipment, and can be utilized in both large and small hospitals as well as at home. A rapid and relatively long-lasting anesthetic effect is produced by 0.5% to 1% lidocaine (Xylocaine) without epinephrine. Local anesthesia is usually more satisfactory if the patient has had some sort of analgesic drug during labor. A combination of Demerol and Phenergan usually produces mental and muscular relaxation as well as analgesia and serves as an excellent premedication.

Local infiltration is the easiest method for peripheral nerve block and is usually quite suitable for spontaneous vaginal delivery and for the performance of episiotomy. A 12.5 cm. narrow-gauge needle is inserted through the skin midway between the anus and the ischial tuberosity, and the anesthetic solution is injected in a fanlike pattern within the area bounded by the tuberosity of the ischium and the descending pubic ramus, the lateral border of the distended vaginal introitus, and the midline of the perineal body. A similar injection is made on the opposite side.

Pudendal nerve block provides more complete anesthesia than does simple local infiltration and is quite adequate for the delivery of most multiparas and many primigravidas. The physician can perform episiotomy and low forceps extraction without difficulty. However, the anesthetic effect usually is inadequate for midforceps delivery or for operative rotation of the head. If pudendal block alone is not adequate, a small amount of nitrous oxide–oxygen with or without Trilene can be administered during the actual delivery. In primigravidas the injection is best made when the presenting part reaches the perineum; however, in multiparas the anesthetic must be given slightly earlier. The necessary manipulation cannot be performed properly when the head is too deep in the pelvis.

DELIVERY

Whether the delivery is accomplished with the patient in the lithotomy position, dorsal position, or lateral position is a matter of personal choice. However, most obstetricians prefer the lithotomy position, even though it does place the perineal structures under unusual tension, because the necessary manipulations are easier and contamination can be prevented better. The lithotomy position is certainly preferable for all operative vaginal deliveries and for the performance of episiotomy. However, the dorsal or lateral position is more comfortable for the patient and quite adequate for spontaneous delivery of multiparas, particularly those with relaxed musculature in whom episiotomy is not necessary and lacerations are not likely to occur. If the lithotomy position is to be used, the lower part of the table should never be removed until the physician is gowned, gloved, and ready to proceed; occasionally, the infant is propelled from the birth canal during an intense uterine contraction, and fatal injury may be sustained if he falls to the floor, whereas little damage will occur if he is born on the cushioned delivery table.

When the physician is properly prepared, the patient's feet are elevated, and she is pulled toward the foot of the table until her buttocks extend

11

slightly over the edge when the lower half of the table is removed. The pubic area and lower abdomen, the vulva and introitus, and the adjacent thighs are scrubbed with green soap or a detergent solution. No attempt is made to cleanse the vagina, and it is not necessary to apply an antiseptic solution to the skin.

The feet, legs, and lower abdomen are covered with sterile drapes, and a sterile sheet is tucked underneath the buttocks. It is not necessary to cover the anus; a drape in this area becomes contaminated almost at once, and it is better to leave the skin uncovered so that feces, blood, and other discharges can be sponged off as they appear. The bladder is emptied with a sterile rubber catheter, the urine being saved for microscopic examination.

Plate 1

Paracervical, or uterosacral, block

Pain sensation from the uterine fundus, the cervix, and the upper vagina is transmitted by way of sympathetic nerve fibers. The route is through the superior hypogastric plexus, which lies anterior to the lumbar vertebras near the bifurcation of the abdominal aorta. The nerves continue downward, dividing into right and left hypogastric branches at the upper sacrum, and approach the uterus along the course of the uterosacral ligaments; they form the *inferior hypogastric plexus* near the uterus on each side. Continuing fibers supply the rectum, uterus, vagina, and bladder.

Transmission of sensation through the inferior hypogastric plexus can be blocked by injecting an anesthetic agent around it. In a successful block, the pain associated with uterine contractions is eliminated. Local infiltration of the perineum or pudendal block is necessary for delivery, since only the upper vagina is anesthetized by paracervical block.

The initial injection is made when the cervix is dilated 4 to 6 cm.; if labor is progressing rapidly, as it may in multiparas, the injection can be made earlier. Ten milliliters of 0.5% to 1% lidocaine are injected between three and four o'clock and between eight and nine o'clock in the vaginal fornices. It is essential that the injection be made superficially enough to raise a wheal; if it is too deep, it will be ineffective. The use of a guide, such as the Iowa trumpet, will ensure proper placement of the tip of the needle. The latter should be long enough to permit its tip to protrude about 5 mm. beyond the end of the guide. The tip of the guide is placed against the fornix and held in place by the index or second finger, the needle is inserted through it until the mucosa is punctured, and the agent is injected.

Plate 1

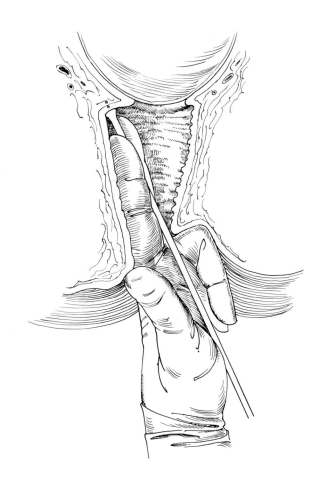

Pain relief occurs promptly, and a single injection usually lasts thirty to forty-five minutes. The injections can be repeated as necessary.

Contractions often slow perceptibly for several minutes after the injection, but when they are reestablished labor progresses at a normal rate.

Fetal bradycardia, probably caused by the absorption of the anesthetic agent into the fetal circulation, occurs frequently. Consequently, this technic should not be used when there is a risk of fetal hypoxia.

13

Plate 2

Conduction anesthesia

The sites of injection for the various types of conduction anesthesia are as follows.

Saddle block (low spinal anesthesia). The needle is introduced into the subarachnoid space between the third and fourth lumbar vertebras while the patient sits on the delivery table with her feet hanging over the side and her spine flexed. If a 26-gauge spinal puncture needle is used, the incidence of postspinal headache can be kept to a minimum. With the small needle it is necessary first to insert a larger introducer between the vertebral bodies to the ligamentum flavum; the dural puncture is made through this introducer. Three to 5 mg. tetracaine (Pontocaine) in 10% dextrose is injected, and the patient remains upright for twenty-five seconds and is then placed flat on her back with her head elevated.

Caudal block. The anesthetic agent to produce caudal anesthesia is introduced extradurally through a needle or catheter that has been introduced into the sacral canal through the caudal hiatus. It is essential to make certain that the needle has not perforated the dura, because the large amount of anesthetic agent will produce massive spinal block if it is injected into the subarachnoid space.

Caudal block eliminates only sensation, in contrast to spinal anesthesia, with which voluntary muscles are paralyzed. The patient can move freely with the caudal block.

Pudendal block. Pain sensations from the perineum, vulva, and lower vagina are eliminated by blocking the pudendal nerve trunk as it passes through Alcock's canal.

Infiltration of perineum. Pain sensation can also be eliminated by anesthetizing the individual peripheral nerve branches arising from the pudendal nerve trunk. This may be quite satisfactory for performance of episiotomy and for spontaneous delivery, but it is less effective than a good pudendal nerve block.

Paracervical block. The inferior hypogastric plexus, through which pain sensation from the uterus, the cervix, and the upper vagina is transmitted, can be blocked by injecting an anesthetic agent through each of the lateral vaginal fornices. Paracervical block must be supplemented to anesthetize the lower vagina and perineum.

14

Plate 2

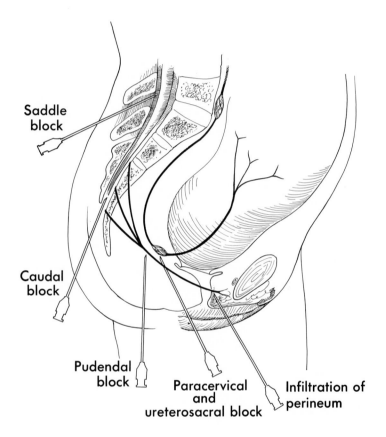

Saddle
block

Caudal
block

Pudendal
block

Paracervical
and
ureterosacral block

Infiltration of
perineum

Plate 3

Pudendal nerve block

A. The pudendal nerve, which is derived from branches of the second, third, and fourth sacral nerves, passes through the greater sciatic foramen and downward to a position behind the ischial spine, where it lies medially to the internal pudendal artery. It continues downward and branches to supply the vulva and perineum. The major peripheral branches are the *inferior rectal (hemorrhoidal) nerve* which supplies the external sphincter, the perianal skin, and the lower anal canal; the *perineal nerve* branches, which supply the labia majora and extend toward the mons pubis, and a deeper branch of which supplies the superficial transverse perineus and the bulbocavernosus and ischiocavernosus muscles; and the *dorsal nerve of the clitoris,* which is deep and which supplies the muscles in the urogenital diaphragm and ends at the clitoris.

When the pudendal nerve trunk is blocked, painful sensations are eliminated from the areas it supplies and the external sphincter and the other voluntary muscles are relaxed.

B. Landmarks for injecting the pudendal nerve trunk. The ischial spine is at the apex of a triangle formed by the sacrospinous and sacrotuberous ligaments and the obturator internus muscle.

C. Injection. The tip of a guide, such as the Iowa trumpet, is directed to a position just beneath the tip of the ischial spine by the index finger and is held firmly in place. A needle at least 12 cm. long is inserted through the guide and into Alcock's canal, through which the nerve trunk runs. After aspirating to be certain that the needle tip does not lie within the pudendal artery or vein, 10 ml. of the anesthetic agent is injected. If blood is withdrawn, the needle is pulled back until it is out of the vessel and the agent is injected. The nerve on the opposite side is then injected.

Anesthesia develops rapidly and should be evident within two or three minutes. The effect can be tested by stroking the skin lateral to the anus with a needle tip; if the anal sphincter does not respond, the nerve has been anesthetized. If the attempt at pudendal block fails on one or both sides, the injection can be repeated.

16

Plate 3

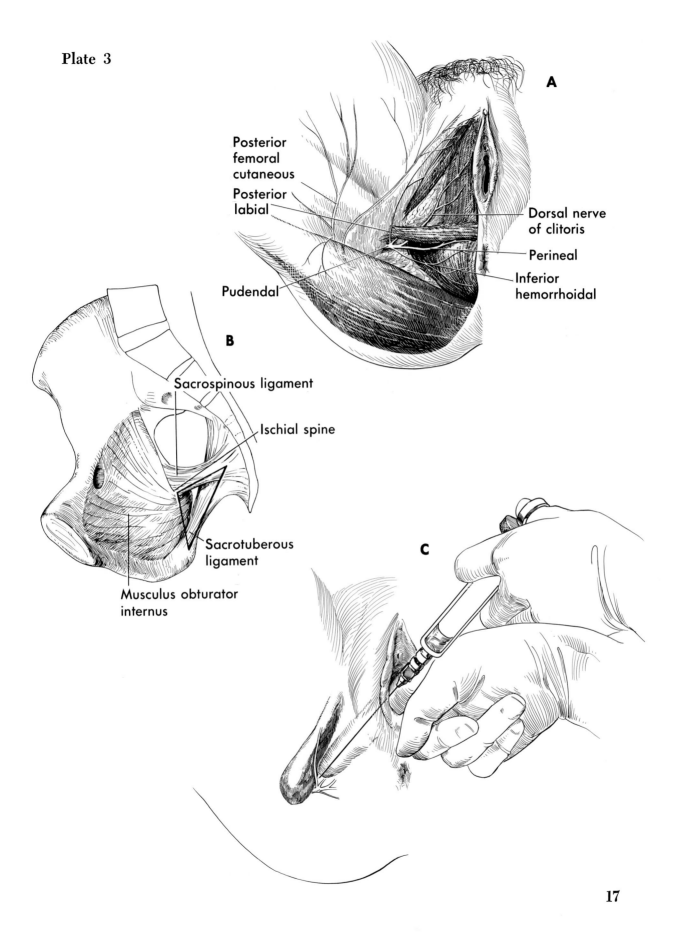

A

Posterior femoral cutaneous

Posterior labial

Pudendal

Dorsal nerve of clitoris

Perineal

Inferior hemorrhoidal

B

Sacrospinous ligament

Ischial spine

Sacrotuberous ligament

Musculus obturator internus

C

17

Plate 4

Normal delivery

A. Position of the head just before normal delivery. The occiput has rotated anteriorly to a position beneath the pubic arch, and the head has descended until it can be seen through the distended introitus during each contraction.

B. Sagittal section showing position of the head.

C. The scalp is visible through the introitus.

D. Vaginal examination is performed to determine the position of the head more accurately. In most instances the posterior fontanel can be readily palpated beneath the pubic arch, with the sagittal suture extending directly posteriorly from it. The anterior fontanel can also be felt, but it may not be easy to reach because the head usually is well flexed.

E. When episiotomy is necessary, it is performed before the muscles and fascial structures have been unduly stretched or torn by the advancing head. Incision also expedites the expulsion of the head by eliminating the barrier of the resisting perineum.

18

Plate 4

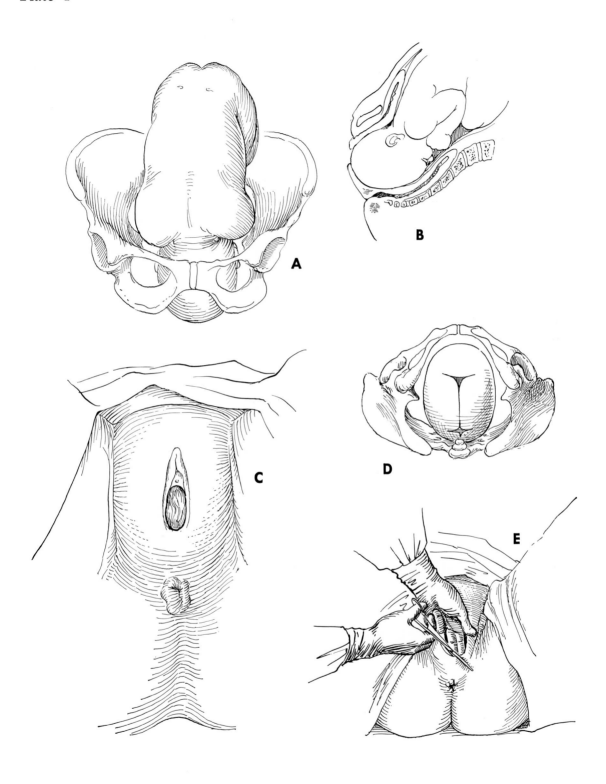

A

B

C

D

E

Plate 4 *Continued*

Normal delivery

F and **G.** With each uterine contraction the infant descends farther through the birth canal until the occipital portion of the head lies beneath the symphysis, where it remains while the forehead and face are pushed upward over the distended perineum as the head extends.

H. Delivery of the head can be assisted by applying upward pressure against the supraorbital ridges with the first and second fingers or with the thumb and index finger. The pressure, which is applied through a sterile towel over the perineum, will maintain extension of the head, thereby preventing it from receding back into the vagina when the uterus relaxes between contractions. The passage of the head through the introitus can be both expedited and controlled by the combination of upward pressure over the forehead to aid extension and descent, and downward pressure on the occiput to resist extension. The proper balance between these two forces permits the obstetrician to deliver the head slowly between uterine contractions, thereby preventing rapid expulsion and possible injury.

I. Extension is now almost complete, and the chin is about ready to clear the perineum, after which the entire head will fall posteriorly.

Plate 4 *Continued*

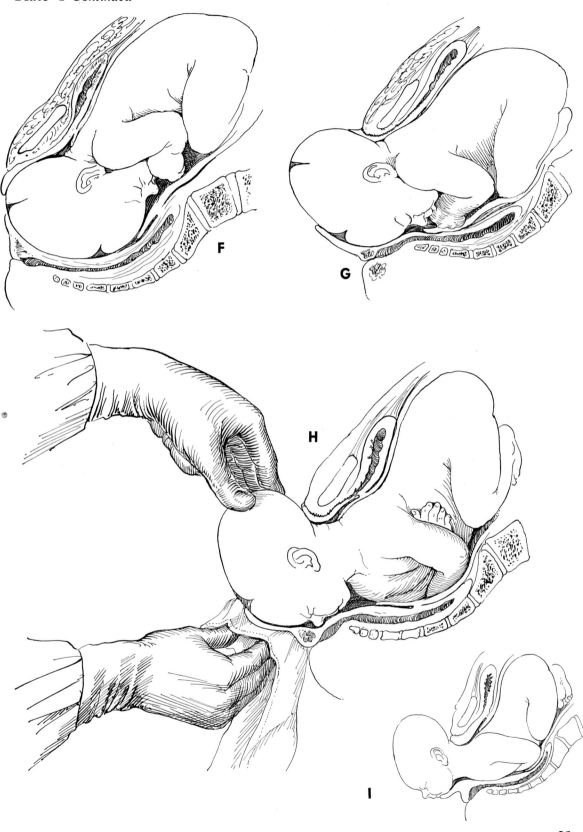

Plate 4 *Continued*

Normal delivery

J. Controlled delivery of the head by balancing upward pressure through the perineum to maintain extension and downward pressure on the occiput to prevent too rapid expulsion.

K. As the eyes and root of the nose appear, the pressure on the occiput can be eliminated, but upward pressure is maintained.

L. The face is delivered by sliding the fingers into the vagina over the infant's cheek and then slipping them beneath the chin, which is gently brought over the perineum.

Plate 4 *Continued*

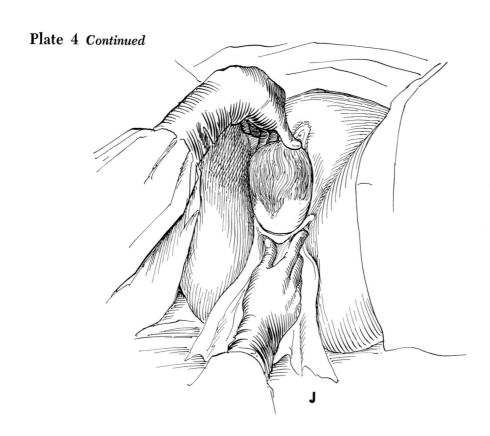

J

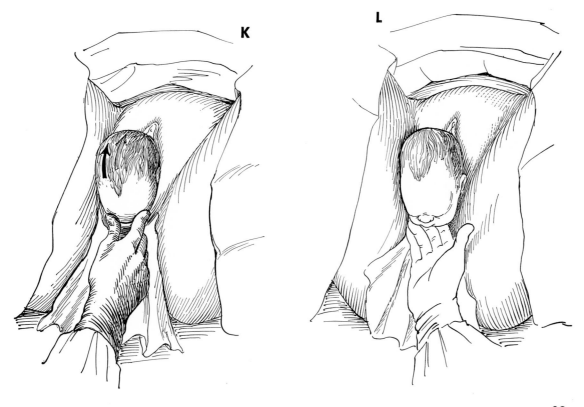

K

L

Plate 4 *Continued*

Normal delivery

M. As uterine contractions continue, the shoulders are forced downward through the inlet in an oblique diameter. With further descent the anterior shoulder rotates to a position behind the symphysis while the posterior shoulder lies below the promontory in the hollow of the sacrum. While the shoulders are descending and rotating, the head is supported in the hands; gentle downward traction may aid descent.

N. Gentle traction in the axis of the birth canal is applied with the hands on each side of the head to produce further descent. The brachial plexus can be injured by too forceful traction. This is particularly true if the anterior shoulder is wedged behind the pubis.

Plate 4 *Continued*

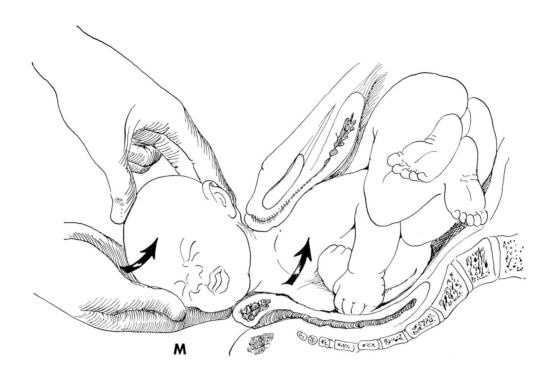

M

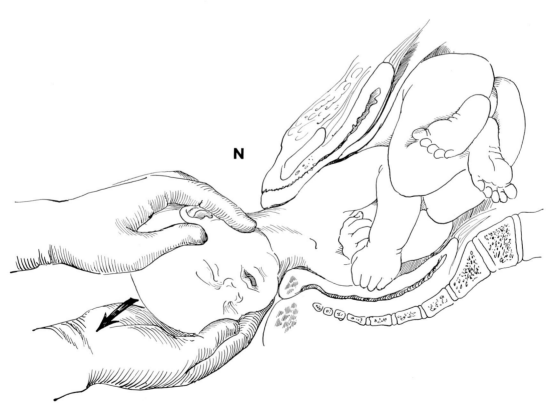

N

Plate 4 *Continued*

Normal delivery

O. Continued traction and depression of the head toward the floor brings the anterior shoulder beneath the symphysis pubis. Traction is maintained until the shoulder and axilla are visible outside the introitus.

P. Too forceful downward traction, particularly if the shoulders are larger than usual, can produce permanent injury to the brachial plexus or even fracture the infant's neck.

Q. The anterior shoulder is allowed to remain in this position for approximately thirty seconds to permit the uterine muscle fibers to retract slightly before the posterior shoulder is delivered. Secretions can be aspirated from the nose and mouth during the waiting period.

Plate 4 *Continued*

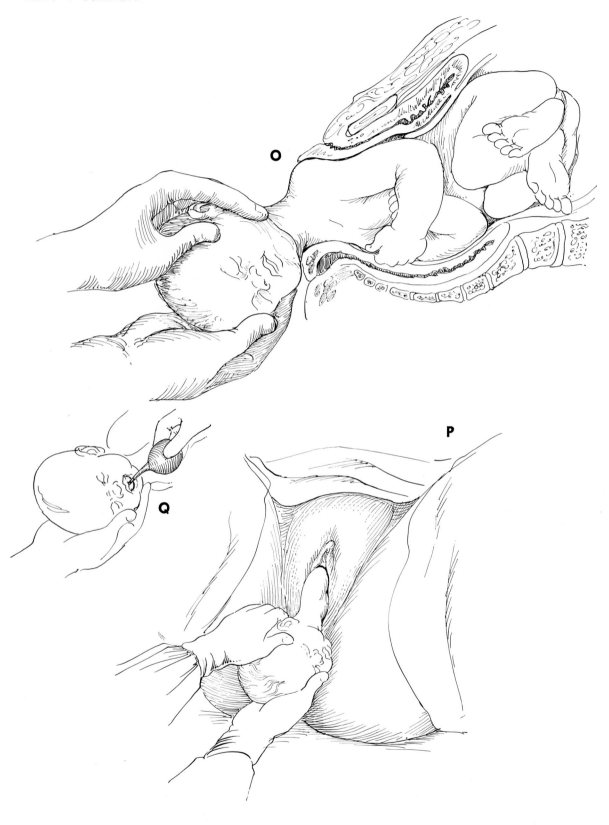

Plate 4 *Continued*

Normal delivery

R. The posterior shoulder is delivered over the perineum by upward traction on the head. After the posterior shoulder has been delivered, further extraction is again delayed for about thirty seconds to permit further retraction of the muscle fibers. However, if the uterus is contracting and forcing the infant downward, no attempt is made to delay the infant's descent.

S. After the second delay, traction is resumed in an outward and upward direction until the axillae have cleared the introitus.

Plate 4 *Continued*

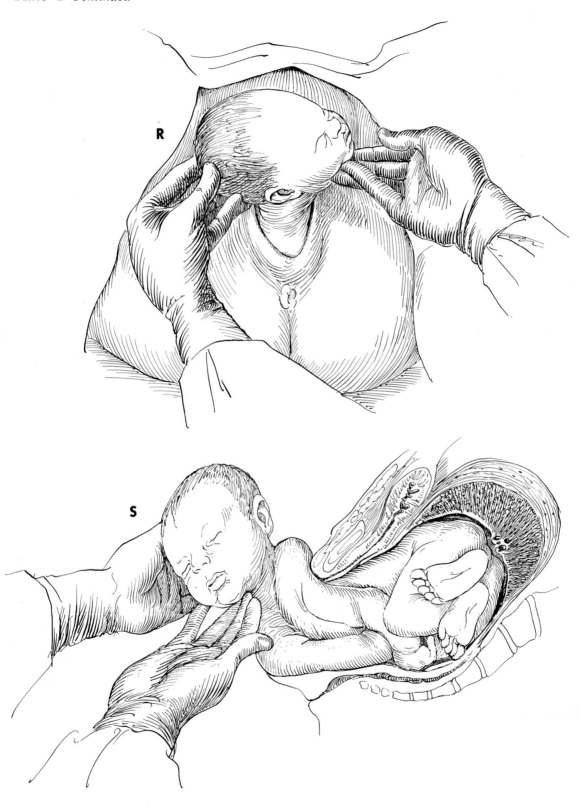

R

S

Plate 4 *Continued*

Normal delivery

T. Further traction is made with the index fingers in the axillae rather than on the head and neck. The head is supported in the left hand.

U. When the umbilicus appears at the introitus, the assistant grasps the cord, pulls a loop downward, and holds it up to prevent contamination from contact with the anus. This will also prevent tension on the umbilical structures as the baby descends if the cord is immobilized between the infant's body and the bony pelvic wall.

Plate 4 *Continued*

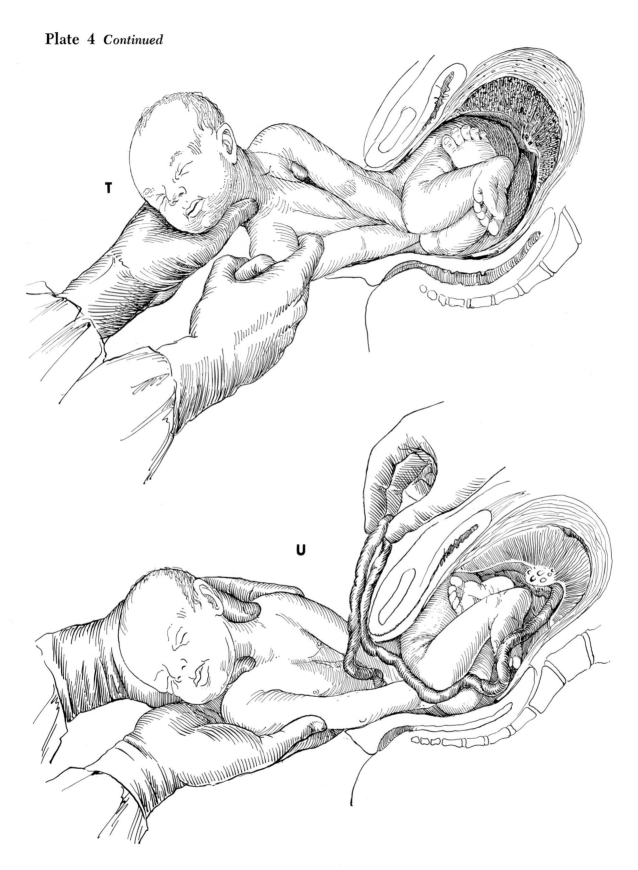

Plate 4 *Continued*

Normal delivery

V. As the baby is slowly extracted, the operator's free hand is slid along the posterior surface of the body until the legs can be grasped at the ankles.

Plate 4 *Continued*

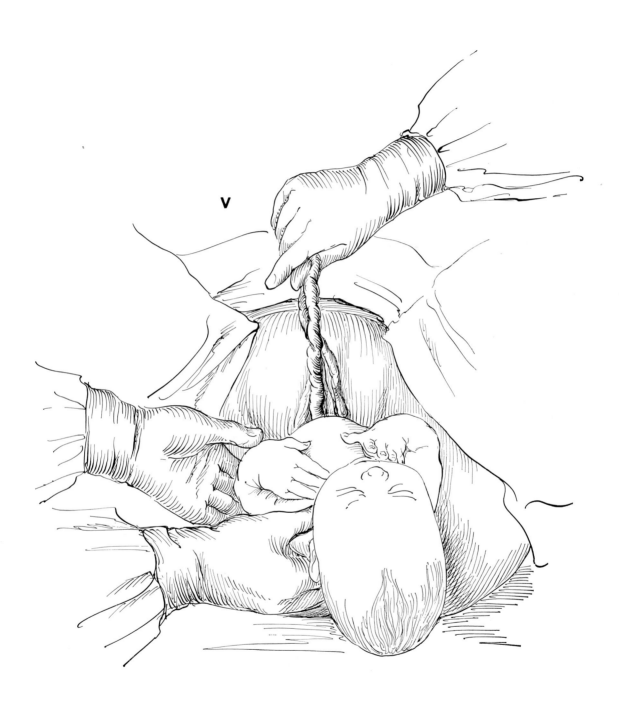

V

Plate 4 *Continued*

Normal delivery

W. The infant is held in an inverted position to aid in draining mucus and secretions from the nasopharynx while an assistant strips the cord from the introitus to the umbilicus several times until the vessels no longer fill with blood. Autotransfusion can also be accomplished by holding the baby below the level of the placenta while the blood drains into his vessels.

X. The cord is severed between the hemostats, and the infant is placed in a warmed crib.

Plate 4 *Continued*

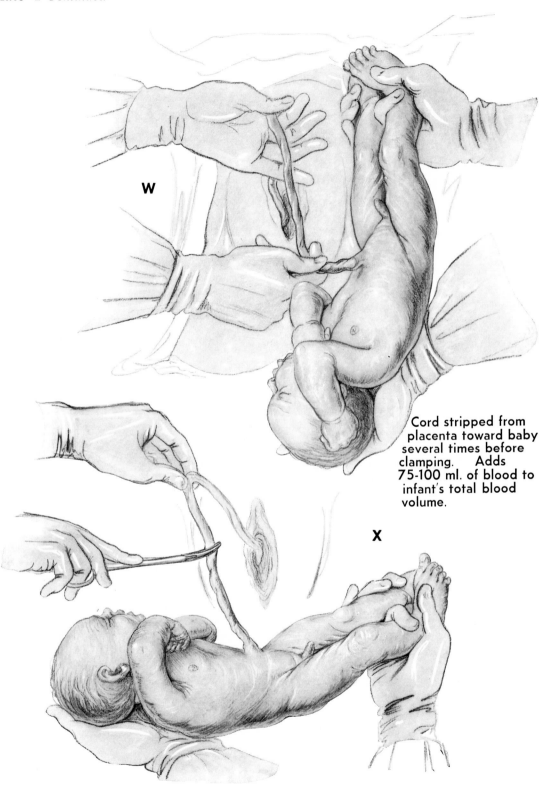

W

Cord stripped from placenta toward baby several times before clamping. Adds 75-100 ml. of blood to infant's total blood volume.

X

Plate 4 *Concluded*

Normal delivery

Y. The cord is occluded by placing a tie, rubber band, or metal clip around it near the skin edge. Before clamping and cutting the cord, one must be certain that there is no herniation of bowel into its proximal portion. This can be suspected if the cord in this area is unusually thick. If the mother is Rh negative, the tie should be placed about 10 cm. from the base of the cord to preserve the vessels in the event exchange transfusion is necessary. If transfusion proves to be unnecessary, the cord can be retied at its base and the distal portion cut off later.

Z. The cord is covered with a dry gauze dressing.

Plate 4 *Concluded*

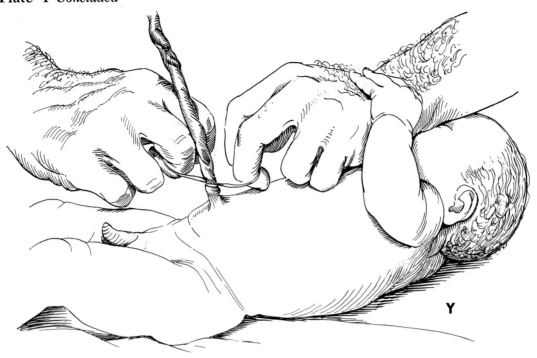

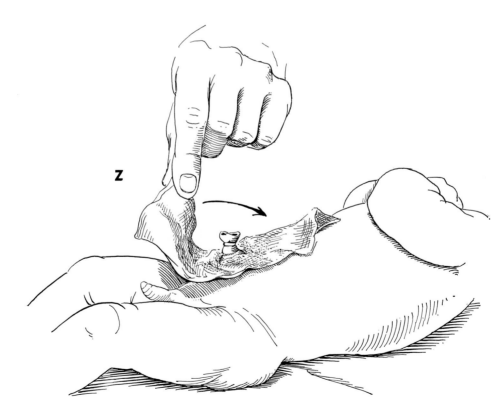

Chapter 3

Shoulder dystocia

If the infant is unusually large or the pelvis of the mother unusually small, the bisacromial diameter may be so great that the shoulders cannot descend through the inlet. Shoulder dystocia can be anticipated whenever cephalopelvic disproportion is encountered or when the infant's head is large and can be extracted from the vagina only with difficulty.

Plate 5

Shoulder dystocia

A. Although the posterior shoulder may lie below the promontory. It can descend no farther until the anterior shoulder slips beneath the pubis; however, this cannot occur because the diameters are so wide. As a result, the neck, which has been stretched by the traction to deliver the head, shortens when the forceps are removed, and the chin is pulled back tightly against the perineum. Unless the delivery is completed, the infant will die of anoxia because the cord is compressed, shutting off the circulation, and the chest cannot yet expand.

B. While the operator exerts downward traction on the head, an assistant applies firm pressure through the abdominal wall on the anterior shoulder in an attempt to push it past the pubis into the pelvis. If this fails, the next maneuver is begun at once.

C. The operator slides his first two fingers, or his entire hand if the shoulder is quite high, into the posterior vagina until his fingertips reach the axilla of the posterior shoulder. If the infant's back is toward the right side of the pelvis, the operator's left hand is used, and if the infant's back is directed toward the left, his right hand is used. An attempt is made to rotate the infant's body 180 degrees and simultaneously to exert traction in the axis of the birth canal.

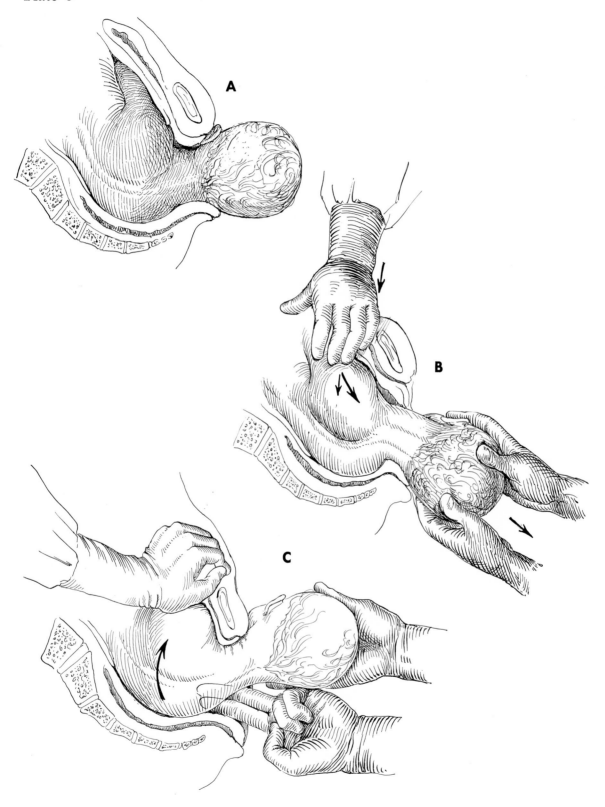

Plate 5

A

B

C

39

Plate 5 *Concluded*

Shoulder dystocia

D. This corkscrew maneuver, if successful, will rotate the anterior shoulder, which was wedged behind the symphysis, into the hollow of the sacrum below the promontory, as the posterior shoulder is being delivered anteriorly. The remainder of the extraction can be accomplished without difficulty. One must take care not to injure the shoulder or fracture the humerus during the rotation.

E. If the shoulders cannot be rotated because they fit so tightly in the pelvis, the bulk of the infant can be reduced by extracting the posterior arm. The operator's fingers or entire hand is inserted into the vagina along the ventral surface of the infant until the infant's hand can be grasped. The baby's hand and forearm are then withdrawn over his chest and past his face. Unless the maneuver is executed carefully, the humerus can be fractured and the shoulder joint injured. This occurs most often if the arm is dragged out posteriorly instead of being flexed over the chest.

F. After the posterior arm has been delivered, it and the posterior shoulder are rotated 180 degrees anteriorly while downward traction is applied. This, as in the previously described maneuver, will not only deliver the shoulder that lay posteriorly but will rotate the impacted anterior shoulder posteriorly into the pelvic cavity, from which it can easily be extracted.

Plate 5 *Concluded*

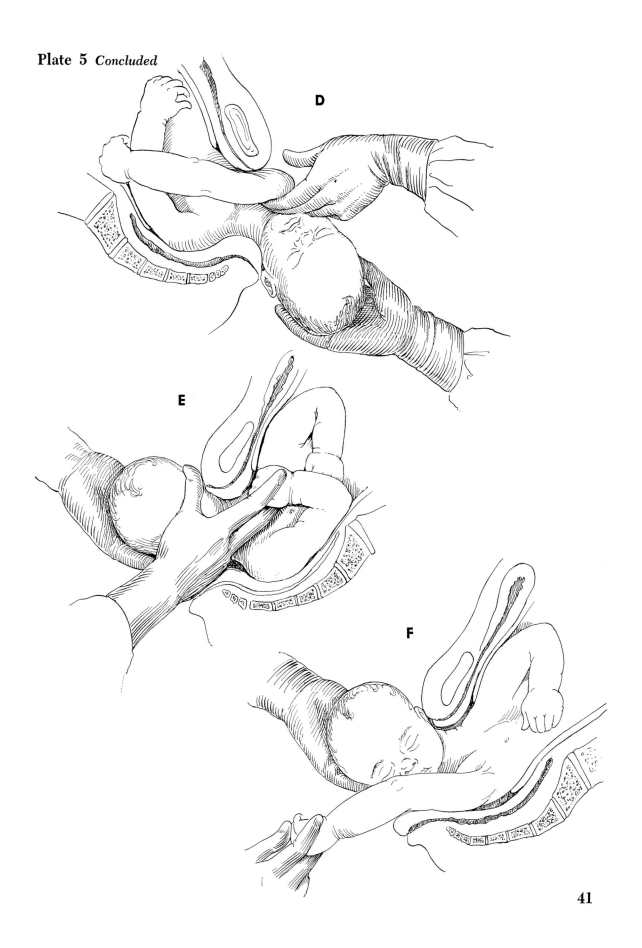

D

E

F

Chapter 4

Third stage of labor and postpartum hemorrhage

THIRD STAGE OF LABOR

Under ordinary circumstances, the placenta will separate from the uterine wall and be extruded from the uterus and vagina without the help of the obstetrician, but the attendant can assist the normal process and thereby shorten the third stage of labor and reduce the blood loss.

The cotyledons of the maternal surface of the placenta extend into the decidua basalis, which forms a natural cleavage plane between the placenta and the uterine wall. The placenta is separated from the decidual attachment by the action of the uterine muscle. The surface area of the uterine cavity gradually increases during pregnancy and rapidly decreases during the second stage of labor. The placenta grows with the placental site during pregnancy, but it has a limited ability to alter its surface area rapidly; therefore it must separate if the area to which it is attached is reduced considerably in size. During pregnancy the area of the placental site probably changes little, even during uterine contractions. This also is true during early labor, because an attached functioning placenta is essential for fetal survival.

As the infant is gradually expelled from the uterus, the cavity must become progressively smaller to permit the uterine wall to remain closely approximated to the infant, thereby maintaining the expulsive force of the muscular contractions. This is accomplished by slight shortening, or retraction, of individual muscle fibers each time a contraction forces the infant a bit farther down the birth canal. The gradual diminution in surface area of the interior of the uterus slightly reduces the diameters of the placental site, and to compensate, the placenta becomes thicker and decreases slightly in diameter. After the birth of the baby, the size of the placenta cannot be reduced as much as the area to which it is attached; it must of necessity separate from the uterine wall. The separation, which occurs in the spongy layer of the decidua basalis, begins during the late second stage of labor and usually is completed as the uterus contracts during the final expulsion of the baby. The effectiveness of the mechanism is determined by the extent to which the placental site area is reduced. If the contractions are firm and forceful, the placenta may be expelled almost immediately after the baby is born; however, if they are less effective, complete placental separation may be delayed.

The blood sinuses at the placental site, which have been opened by partial or complete separation of the placenta, are the source of bleeding during and after the third stage of normal labor. Bleeding from the sinuses is controlled initially by firm contraction of the interlacing uterine muscle bundles around the branches of the uterine arteries that course through the wall to the placental area. If the muscle contracts normally, the vessels are compressed and kinked, and bleeding from the open ends is slight, but if the uterus is relaxed, fatal hemorrhage will occur. Blood loss during the third stage of labor can usually be reduced if the possibility of muscular atony is recognized or anticipated and preventive measures are initiated. The prevention and treatment of prolonged and dysfunctional labor by artificial rupture of membranes, administration of intravenous fluids, and judicious use of oxytocics will aid in correcting inertia and the resultant abnormal bleeding. Slow delivery of the shoulders and body of the infant will permit the muscle fibers to retract and adjust to the reduction in size of the cavity, thereby promoting more efficient contraction. Of at least equal importance is the meticulous management of the third stage of labor by an obstetrician who understands the methods by which the normal separation and expulsion of the placenta can be expedited.

Blood loss can be reduced by the administration of uterotonic drugs to promote muscle contraction after the delivery of the placenta. Some obstetricians give a drug intravenously when the anterior shoulder is delivered beneath the pubis. It will then reach and stimulate the uterine muscle at about the time the baby is delivered, and if the timing is correct, the placenta will often emerge with the baby. Most obstetricians prefer to administer the drugs immediately after the delivery of the placenta. Oxytocin, 2 units, ergonovine malleate (Ergotrate), 0.2 mg., or methylergonovine tartrate (Methergine), 0.2 mg., may be injected intravenously at the end of the third stage. Oxytocin, 10 units, or 0.2 mg. of the ergot compounds can be injected intramuscularly after placental delivery. The onset of action is slightly slower than after intravenous injection, but this route is quite appropriate for normal patients.

POSTPARTUM HEMORRHAGE

Postpartum hemorrhage, a blood loss greater than 500 ml., does occur from time to time, but death can almost always be avoided if adequate preventive and therapeutic measures are utilized. Excessive bleeding can be expected to occur whenever uterine muscle activity is decreased. The physician must be prepared to treat postpartum hemorrhage if the contractions are weak and relatively ineffectual because of dysfunctional labor or because of overdistention caused by multiple pregnancy or polyhydramnios, or if they must be abolished by anesthesia for an operative delivery, such as version or breech extraction.

Excessive bleeding in the third stage of labor almost always originates at the placental site rather than from an injury and can therefore be controlled if firm uterine contractions can be stimulated by administering an oxytocic, by manually elevating and massaging the uterus, and by removing portions of retained placenta and blood clots from the cavity. No time should be wasted in attempts to inspect the cervix and vagina for injury unless the uterus is firmly contracted, in which event the bleeding may be from a laceration.

While the uterus is elevated and massaged between the hand in the vagina and the other palpating through the abdominal wall, 0.2 mg. Methergine or 0.2 mg. Ergotrate is given intravenously. If the uterus does not contract promptly, the cavity is explored by careful manual palpation in an attempt to locate a fragment of adherent placenta, a traumatic defect in the wall, or some other abnormality. A repeat injection of Ergotrate or Methergine can be administered, but if the uterus remains soft in spite of the measures already utilized, a continuous drip of dilute oxytocin solution (1:1000) may prove more effective.

Intrauterine packs have been used extensively in the past to control postpartum hemorrhage, but the resultant distention of the uterus may increase rather than stop bleeding. If bleeding continues despite the packing, another method for control should be instituted. Removal and replacement of the pack will almost always be ineffectual and will only delay the application of effective treatment and increase the total blood loss.

When all other measures fail, the physician has no choice but to remove the uterus, but before a final decision is made, the clotting mechanism should be studied. Occasionally, persistent bleeding may be a result of hypofibrinogenemia, which can be corrected by the administration of fibrinogen, or of some other disturbance in the clotting mechanism. To determine the coagulation time, 10 ml. of venous blood is placed in a clean test tube and observed for clotting. If a firm clot forms promptly and subsequently retracts well, the coagulation mechanism is intact. If the blood fails to clot or if a soft clot forms but is lysed promptly, a clotting defect can be suspected.

Successful treatment of serious postpartum hemorrhage depends, in a large measure, upon adequate blood replacement. Blood transfusion should be started early and continued until bleeding is controlled and the pulse and blood pressure are stable. Sudden overwhelming postpartum hemorrhage almost never occurs. In almost every instance the bleeding is moderate but persistent and can be controlled if appropriate diagnostic and therapeutic measures are instituted and if the lost blood is replaced.

Plate 6

Delivery of the placenta

A. During the birth of the infant, the placenta is at least partially separated from its attachment to the uterine wall, but it will remain within the cavity while the muscle fibers gradually shorten until they can contract effectively enough to complete the third stage of labor. The placental site is usually located on either the anterior or the posterior wall; consequently, the relaxed uterus is flattened in its anteroposterior diameter but is widened transversely. The shape of the uterus can be determined by abdominal palpation, but no attempt should be made to massage or manipulate it at this time because artificially produced contractions may disturb the normal mechanism and delay placental separation.

B. During a uterine contraction, the flattened body becomes globular as the placenta is forced downward into the lower segment. Expulsion of the placenta from the upper segment can be assisted by firm pressure over the fundus in the axis of the birth canal. It is not necessary to squeeze the uterus between the thumb and fingers.

C. As the placenta leaves the upper part of the uterus, the uterus becomes harder and more globular. When this change is felt, the placenta can be forced downward toward the introitus at the same time the uterus is being pushed upward by firm pressure against the lower uterine segment through the abdominal wall. If the placenta is incompletely separated or partially trapped by contraction of the lower border of the upper segment, the cord can be avulsed by excessive traction. Consequently, expulsive pressure is applied from above rather than by traction on the funis.

D. The third stage of labor is completed by pushing the uterus upward out of the pelvis and away from the placenta by firm pressure with the fingertips of the abdominal hand while downward traction is exerted on the cord to guide the placenta through the vagina and to keep it from following the uterus upward.

46

Plate 6

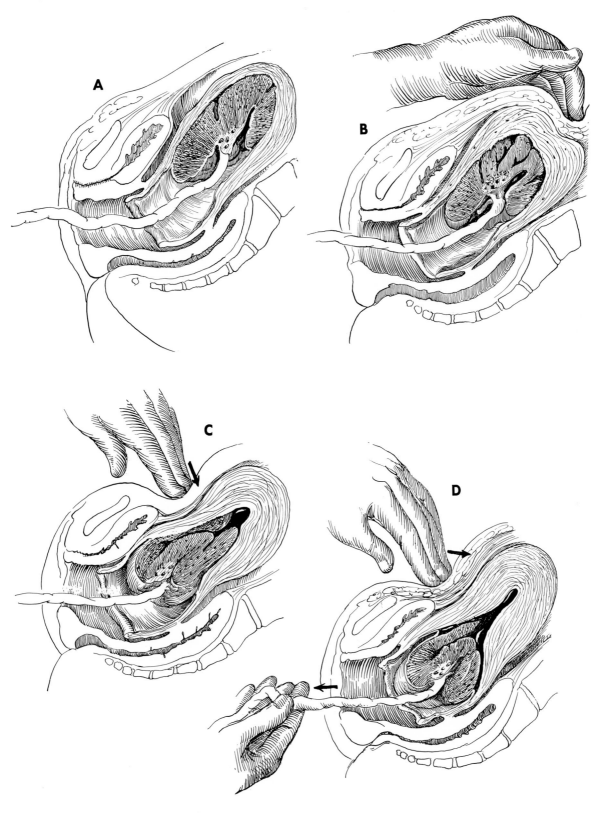

47

Plate 6 *Concluded*

Delivery of the placenta

E. The placenta is caught in a large sterile basin as it is expressed from the vagina.

F. As the uterus is pushed upward by pressure on the fundus through the abdominal wall, the trailing membranes that may adhere slightly to the uterine walls are teased off by gentle traction with hemostats applied successively one above the other as more of the amnion appears.

G. The adherent membranes are being pulled off the lower segment.

Plate 6 *Concluded*

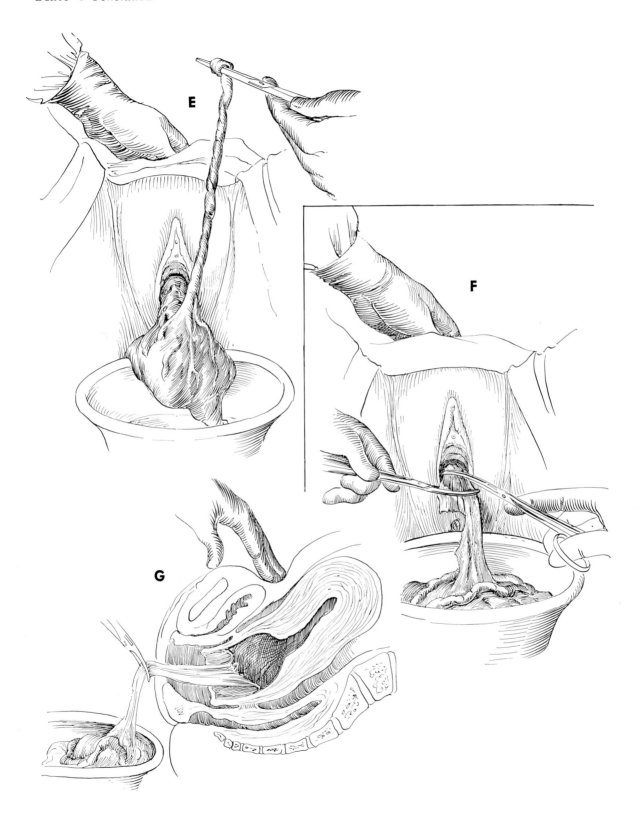

Plate 7

Manual removal of the placenta

Manual removal of the placenta becomes necessary whenever the normal mechanism for expulsion fails or when bleeding is profuse and it is impossible to complete the third stage of labor by the usual external manipulations. Properly performed manual removal is not dangerous; it fact, when done for bleeding, it should decrease morbidity and mortality.

The third stage of labor usually is completed within five minutes, but it may be unduly prolonged either because the placenta is abnormally adherent (placenta accreta) or because the uterine muscle beneath the placental site is relaxed and boggy, preventing separation, even though the muscle in the rest of the uterus is fairly well contracted. No bleeding can occur as long as the placenta remains completely attached, but profuse hemorrhage from the open sinuses may follow its partial separation. The bleeding will continue as long as the placenta remains in the uterus, preventing the firm contraction necessary to occlude the vessels terminating in the open placental site sinuses.

The placenta should be removed promptly if bleeding is excessive and if it cannot be expressed by the usual manipulations. If no bleeding occurs, the obstetrician may await spontaneous separation and expulsion, but there is no reason for waiting more than five to ten minutes before invading the cavity. The patient should remain in the delivery room until the placenta is delivered, and facilities for transfusion and operation must be immediately available in the event that the placenta is abnormally adherent and attempts to remove it cause excessive hemorrhage.

The cotyledons of a *placenta accreta* invade the uterine muscle directly because the decidua basalis layer is absent. As a result there is no cleavage plane, and separation of the invasive area is impossible. If the entire surface of the placenta is adherent, no bleeding can occur. However, hemorrhage may be profuse if part of the placenta is normally implanted and can be detached and the remainder cannot, because it will be impossible to empty the uterus to permit it to contract. Unless the area of abnormal implantation is small, hysterectomy is usually indicated.

Manual removal of the placenta should never be performed in home deliveries except to control hemorrhage. It is not usually necessary to pack the uterus after the placenta has been removed, and antibiotics need not be ordered.

Plate 7

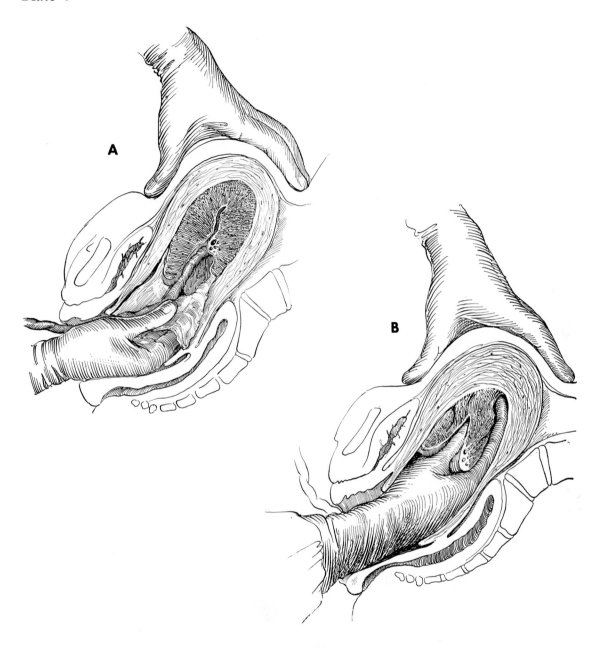

A. After the operator changes his gloves, cleanses the vulva, and applies clean drapes, he inserts his hand through the cervix between the uterine wall and the amniotic membrane until he can feel the edge of the placenta. He steadies the uterus with his other hand by holding the fundus through the abdominal wall.

B. The cleavage plane in the decidua basalis is located and the placenta is separated by sweeping the extended fingers back and forth between it and the uterus until the afterbirth is completely free and can be grasped and withdrawn. The operator then reinserts his hand and palpates the entire cavity with his fingertips, searching for remaining fragments of placental tissue.

Plate 7 *Concluded*

Manual removal of the placenta

C. If most of the placenta is implanted anteriorly, it often can be separated most easily if the palmar surface of the hand is directed anteriorly. After separation is complete, the hand can be pronated to permit its grasping and extracting the freed placenta.

D. The palmar surface of the hand is upward while the placenta is being separated from the anterior wall.

Plate 7 *Concluded*

C

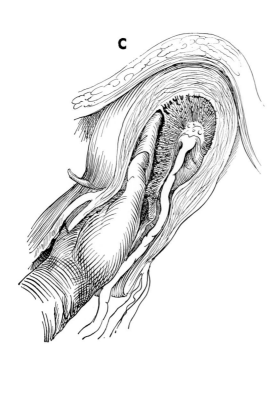

D

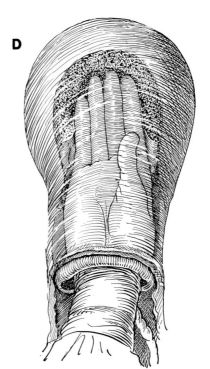

Plate 8

Removal of the placental fragments and insertion of the uterine pack

A. After the vulvar area is cleansed, the operator's hand is passed into the uterus and the entire surface of the cavity is palpated. Adherent fragments of placenta are scraped off the placental site with his fingertips. When the uterus is empty, it is elevated and massaged between one hand, which is in the vagina, and the other hand palpating through the abdominal wall. An oxytocic is administered intravenously at this time.

B. The operator's left hand is passed through the cervix, with the palmar surface directed anteriorly, and the uterine pack is inserted into the upper segment while the uterus is steadied by an assistant, who holds the fundus through the abdominal wall.

Plate 8

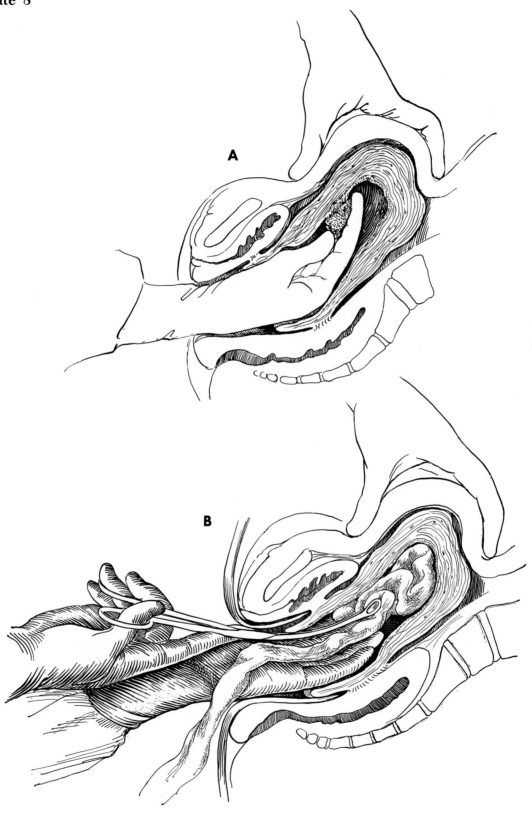

A

B

Plate 8 *Concluded*

Removal of the placental fragments and insertion of the uterine pack

C. The operator forces the packing upward against the fundus and distributes it throughout the upper part of the uterus in order to make certain that the entire cavity is filled.

D. Packing is continued systematically until the entire uterovaginal cavity is firmly occluded.

E. If only the lower segment of the uterus and the vagina are packed, blood from the placental sinuses may accumulate in the upper segment. This may not be detected until the pack is saturated and blood begins to drip from the introitus.

Plate 8 *Concluded*

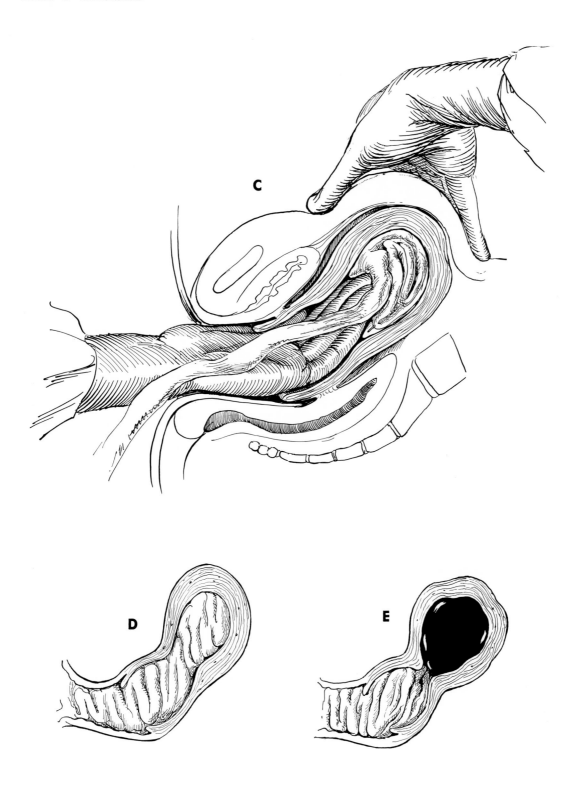

Inversion of the uterus

On rare occasions the uterus will invert and prolapse through the cervical opening during or immediately after the delivery of an infant. The cause is not always obvious, but in most instances the placenta is implanted over the most superior surface of the uterus rather than on the anterior or posterior wall of the cavity. The weight of the placenta pulls the relaxed uterine fundus downward into the flaccid lower segment after the baby is expelled, and the next uterine contraction forces the fundus and placenta through the dilated cervix; the fundus and placenta may also be pulled down by injudicious traction on the cord. Inversion is *complete* if the uterus is turned completely inside out and *partial* if only a portion of it protrudes through the cervical opening. In the former the fundus and the attached placenta usually descend through the introitus, whereas in the incomplete varieties the inverted uterus may not be visible although it lies in the vagina.

Complete inversion usually is obvious because the fundus of the uterus can be seen outside the introitus, and partial inversion can easily be detected even though the placenta appeared to have delivered normally. When the physician attempts to palpate the uterus above the pubis, he feels a depression rather than a firmly contracted globular mass, and the inverted fundus can be felt by vaginal palpation or seen when the cervix and vagina are inspected.

Since profuse bleeding and shock usually occur after the placenta separates, prompt recognition and treatment are essential. Intravenous administration of saline solution should be started in order that blood may be administered promptly if profuse bleeding occurs. If bleeding is not excessive and the inversion is not recognized, the fundus may become incarcerated by the constricting collar of muscle, making replacement much more difficult.

Plate 9

Management of acute inversion

A. The placenta is separated from the protruding fundus in the cleavage plane of the decidua basalis.

Plate 9

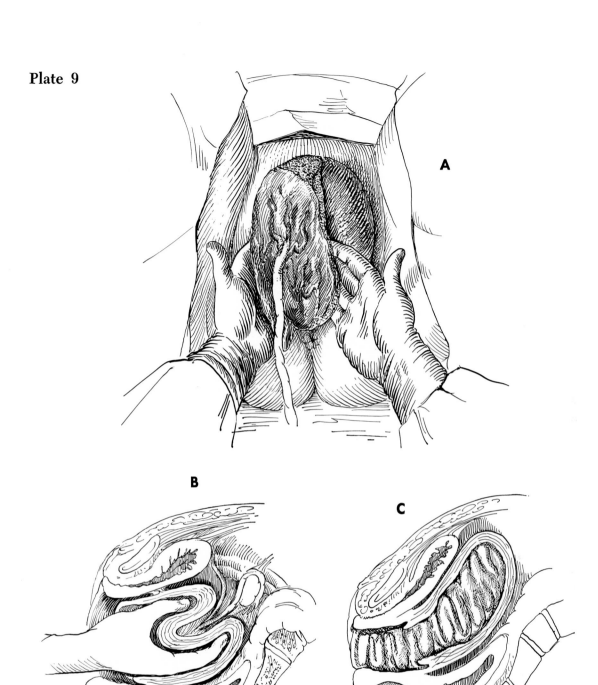

B. The inverted uterus is grasped in the operator's entire hand, with the fundus resting on the palmar surface and the fingertips exerting equal pressure around the collar of the uterus within the cervical opening. The fundus is replaced with upward pressure. Replacement usually is not difficult if the inversion is corrected before the uterus contracts firmly.

C. Before the hand is removed from the uterine cavity, a tight uterovaginal pack is inserted. This can be removed after twenty-four hours—first withdrawing the vaginal portion and later the portion in the uterine cavity.

Plate 10

Management of chronic inversion

Chronic inversion is more difficult to correct because of uterine muscle contraction, which constricts the opening through which the fundus has prolapsed. It usually is necessary to incise the constricting collar of muscle before the uterus can be replaced. In most instances, this is best accomplished through an abdominal rather than a vaginal approach.

A. The uterus is completely inverted, with the fundal portions of the tubes and round ligaments pulled downward through the constricting collar. A malleable retractor is placed in the posterior vagina, with its tip inserted between the posterior lip of the cervix and the inverted uterine wall at the point at which the muscle will be cut.

Plate 10

A

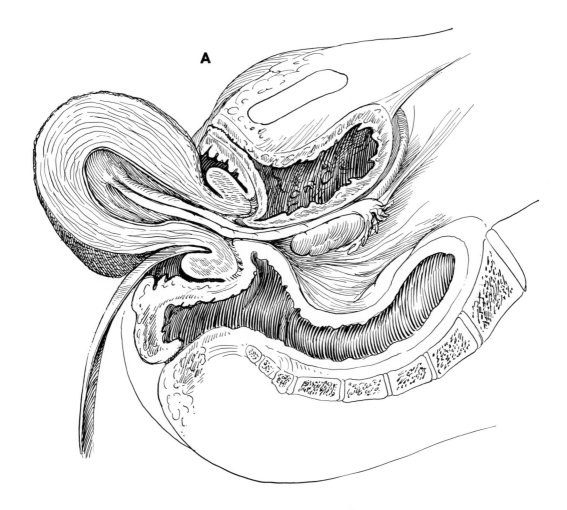

Plate 10 *Concluded*

Management of chronic inversion

B. The rectosigmoid is held out of the way while an incision is made entirely through the uterine wall at the point of greatest constriction. The length of the incision will vary but should be long enough to permit passage of the fundus. If the incision is made over the previously placed malleable retractor, only the uterus will be incised, and the vaginal structures will not be injured.

C. The fundus is replaced by combined traction on the uterine wall from above by the operator and pressure from below by an assistant. When replacement is complete, the incision is closed with interrupted catgut sutures. It is not usually necessary to pack the cavity after replacing a chronically inverted uterus. The constricted area that prevented its replacement will also prevent reinversion. An intrauterine pack will also increase morbidity, since the endometrial surface of a chronically inverted uterus always is heavily infected.

Plate 10 *Concluded*

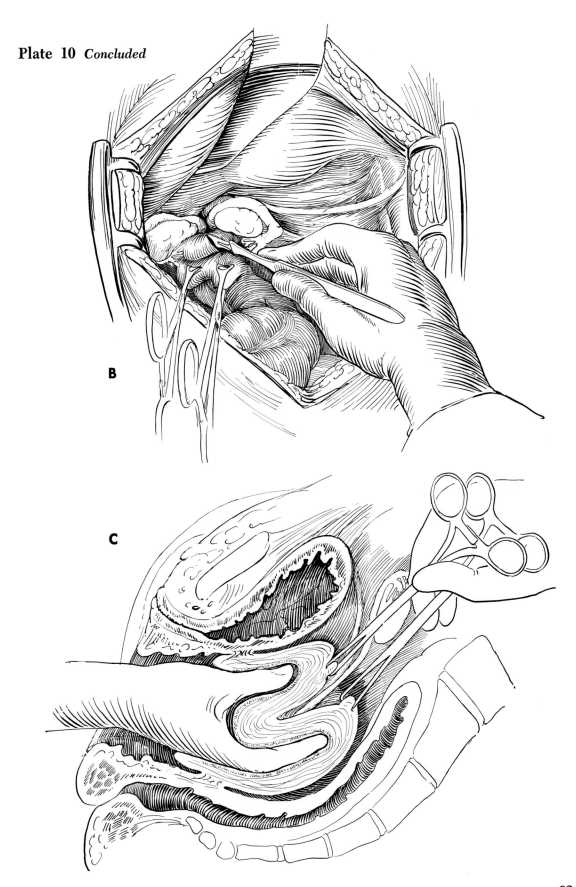

B

C

Chapter 5

Induction of labor

Although the artificial induction of labor has become increasingly popular in recent years, it is not often necessary for normal women; in fact, under certain circumstances, the risk to both mother and infant may be increased by the procedure. Termination of pregnancy, however, may play an important part in the management of certain complications, particularly those accompanied by bleeding and in patients with one of the toxemias.

INDICATIONS

Toxemia. Most indicated inductions will be performed in women with one of the toxemias of pregnancy. Delivery of a patient with advancing severe preeclampsia that cannot be controlled with medical treatment may prevent the development of eclampsia, with its resultant high maternal and infant mortality. The same holds true for the delivery of a patient with acute toxemia superimposed on chronic hypertension.

Bleeding. Rupture of membranes in certain patients with incomplete placenta previa may control bleeding by permitting the presenting part to descend and compress the separated area of placenta against the uterine wall; in addition, it will permit vaginal delivery. The disadvantage of vaginal delivery is that the total area of placenta eliminated by separation and compression may be so great that the fetus cannot survive. As a consequence, cesarean section is usually preferable to induction if the baby has a reasonable chance of surviving when delivery becomes necessary. On the other hand, induction and vaginal delivery usually are preferable to cesarean section when the infant is dead or is so premature that it has little chance to survive, as long as the procedure does not add greatly to the risk for the mother. Induction is often feasible for patients with either mild or severe abruptio placentae. Profuse bleeding is not necessarily a contra-indication to vaginal delivery, because hemorrhage with premature separation so often is caused by hypofibrinogenemia, which can be corrected by the administration of fibrinogen.

Ruptured membranes. If labor does not begin spontaneously within twelve hours after rupture of the membranes, oxytocin stimulation can be considered. Induction is probably more important for premature infants than for those near term because the death rate from infection, which is increased with ruptured membranes, is far higher in smaller infants than in those which are more mature.

Fetal indications. In an occasional patient the fetus dies in utero during the last few weeks of successive pregnancies. Under these circumstances, termination of pregnancy by induction before the infant expires may permit the birth of a normal baby. Early induction may be indicated in patients with metabolic disorders, such as diabetes, if babies have been born dead or seriously ill in previous pregnancies. However, in many women with diabetes, the best infant survival rate is obtained by delivery at about thirty-six weeks, when induction is not feasible; consequently, cesarean section is often more practical. The repeated measurement of the daily urinary estriol excretion is helpful in determining the proper time for delivery of a mother with diabetes. A falling or abnormally low level suggests that the baby should be delivered regardless of the duration of pregnancy. Early delivery may also be indicated when several infants have died in utero with erythroblastosis, but induction should not be considered simply because the mother is sensitized. The severity of fetal involvement, which can be assessed by serial determination of the optical density of amniotic fluid during the last trimester, is the essential factor in evaluating the need for delivery.

Elective induction. Elective induction constitutes the most frequent reason for induction in private patients, and when these patients are carefully selected and the procedure is properly performed, it does not add greatly to the risk. It is difficult to justify elective induction on the basis of protection for either the baby or the mother, except in multiparas with uncertain transportation who live some distance from the hospital and who have had rapid labors in the past or in those in whom the cervix is found to be dilated several centimeters during the last few weeks of pregnancy. Elective induction in primigravidas is almost never warranted.

SELECTION OF METHODS AND PATIENTS

Selection of methods. Labor can be induced by rupturing the membranes and draining off the amniotic fluid, by stimulating uterine contractions with an oxytocic substance, or by a combination of the two methods. Voorhees' bags and bougies are less effective than either amniotomy or stimulation and are potentially more dangerous because of the possibility of introducing infecting organisms directly into the uterine cavity. Regardless of which technic is utilized, the best results will be obtained when the patients are carefully selected and when those in whom it is important to terminate pregnancy but who are unsuitable for induction are delivered by cesarean section.

Selection of patients. A decision as to whether or not induction is possible is based upon the condition of the cervix, the position and station of the infant, the parity, and the duration of the pregnancy. As a general rule, the more advanced the pregnancy, the more effective the methods of induction, but the final decision must be based upon the condition of the cervix as determined by vaginal examination rather than upon the history. If the cervix is soft, in the center of the birth canal, and at least partially effaced and dilated 2 or 3 cm. in multiparas and completely effaced with the same dilation in primigravidas, induction will probably be successful. However, if the cervix is firm, posterior, and uneffaced, induction usually is not possible even under the most favorable conditions. It usually is easier to initiate labor in multiparas than in primigravidas.

It is easier and safer to start labor when the infant is in an occiput position than when he is in a breech position, although it is possible in the latter. Induction can rarely be justified if the head is deflexed or with transverse or oblique lies. Of course, the pelvis must be large enough to permit passage of the baby.

Induction of labor is contraindicated unless there is a logical reason for terminating pregnancy and certainly whenever the previously described conditions are not present.

Plate 11

Induction of labor

A. Sterile vaginal examination table containing sterile drape for abdomen, catheter and urine specimen bottle, uterine dressing forceps, Graves' speculum, and solution basins containing sterile soap solution and sterile water.

B. Sterile vaginal examination is performed to determine the position, station, and condition of the cervix and pelvis before any type of induction. Leggings are not necessary, but the abdomen is covered with a sterile sheet after the perineum is prepared with a sterile soap solution. The operator scrubs his hands and forearms and wears sterile gloves, but he does not need to don a sterile gown. The labia are separated to permit introduction of the examining fingers without contamination from the vulvar skin.

Oxytocin induction (medical induction). Stimulation of uterine contractions with dilute oxytocin solution is preferable to artificial rupture of the membranes when the infant's head is not yet engaged or if the infant is presenting in a breech position. However, it is a less certain method than amniotomy, and the potential hazards are greater. Tetanic uterine contractions may reduce blood flow through the placental sinuses, thereby interfering with oxygenation of the infant. If the drug is administered too rapidly, the tumultuous activity of the uterus may drive the infant through the birth canal with such force that both the baby and the maternal soft tissues will suffer serious injury. If there is obstruction to the descent of the fetus, the uterus may rupture; this is particularly likely to occur in women of high parity. Complications can be avoided by proper selection of patients for induction and by careful administration of the oxytocin under constant supervision.

C. An intravenous drip of 5% dextrose is started in one of the veins in the back of the hand or forearm, and the needle is taped in place. The needle leading from a plainly marked flask containing 10 units (1 ml.) of oxytocin in 1000 ml. of 5% dextrose is then inserted into the tubing of the previously started intravenous system.

The rate of flow of the oxytocin-containing solution is best controlled by an infusion pump that will permit precise regulation of the amount of oxytocin being introduced into the system. While the plain dextrose solution is administered at a rate of about 5 drops per minute, enough to keep the needle open, the infusion of oxytocin solution is started at a rate of 2 mμ per minute. If the uterus fails to contract or if only slight activity is induced within ten

67

or fifteen minutes, the rate of flow can be increased to about 5 mμ per minute. The dosage is gradually increased until a pattern of uterine activity like that during normal labor is produced. This can usually be achieved with no more than 10 to 15 mμ per minute if the uterine muscle is sensitive enough for successful induction. The amount of oxytocin administered is determined by the response; it usually is necessary to adjust it from time to time to maintain contractions similar to those which occur during normal labor. After the contractions have been recurring regularly for thirty to sixty minutes, the flow of oxytocin can be slowed or stopped, with the needle remaining in the vein. If labor continues without stimulation, the needle can be removed; however, if the contractions become short and irregular, an effective rate of flow can be reestablished. If the membranes are ruptured artificially after the head has descended farther, labor will usually improve and often will continue without additional stimulation.

When an infusion pump is not available, the flow rate of oxytocin can be varied by opening and closing the clamp leading from the bottle. An initial rate of 5 to 10 drops per minute can gradually be increased until the desired contraction pattern is obtained. The infusion pump provides more accurate and less variable flow than does the drop method.

Since oxytocin induction is hazardous, an experienced observer should remain with the patient to whom the solution is being administered. He should time and palpate uterine contractions, count the fetal heart rate, record maternal blood pressure frequently, and adjust the rate of flow of the solution as necessary. Oxytocin should never be administered unless someone can stay with the patient; if he must leave, the oxytocic drug is discontinued until he returns.

Plate 11

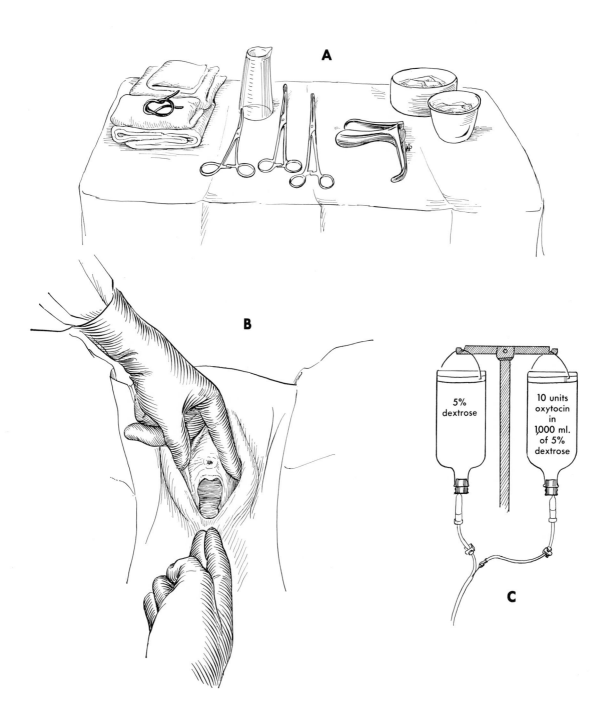

A

B

5% dextrose

10 units oxytocin in 1,000 ml. of 5% dextrose

C

Plate 11 *Concluded*

Induction of labor

Rupture of membranes. Amniotomy is a very effective method for initiating labor, but it is not entirely innocuous even when performed under the best of conditions. The cord or a fetal extremity may be washed through the introitus by the gush of amniotic fluid if an irregular breech presents or if the head has not descended far enough to occlude the pelvic inlet and the cervical opening. Amniotomy as an initial step in the induction of labor, particularly for elective inductions, is usually contraindicated unless the cervix is soft and effaced, the occiput is presenting, and the head is engaged.

D. Sterile vaginal examination is performed to evaluate the cervix and to determine fetal position and station. The fingers are swept around the presenting part inside the cervical opening to separate membranes from the cervix. The head is pushed up slightly to permit fluid to gravitate into the pouching forebag.

E. Uterine dressing forceps or an Allis clamp is introduced along the fingers, and the membranes are grasped and torn. This is best done when the uterus is relaxed, because the cord may be washed out with the gushing fluid if the membranes are perforated during a contraction.

F. The operator can prove that he actually has ruptured the membranes by pulling a tuft of hair from the infant's scalp.

G. Amniotomy is usually more effective if much of the fluid is evacuated from the uterus. If the head is pushed upward slightly and pressure is exerted against the fundus of the uterus with the outside hand, a considerable portion of the fluid can be expressed. The operator need only disengage the head; if it is pushed upward out of the pelvis, the cord or an extremity may prolapse.

Plate 11 *Concluded*

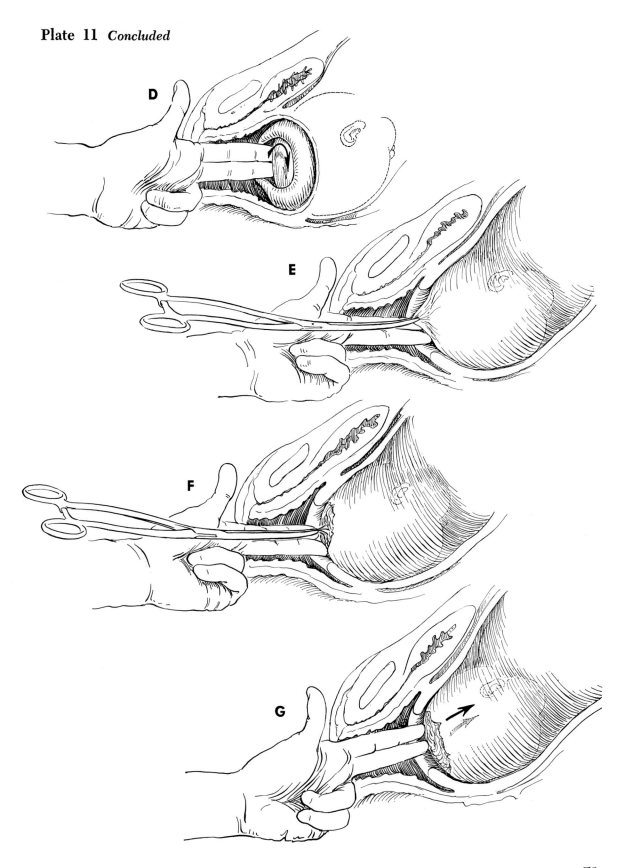

Chapter 6

Prevention and management of childbirth injury

Injury to the soft tissues must almost inevitably occur during delivery unless the structures either are so resilient that they can stretch without tearing or are already thoroughly relaxed from previous damage. In some persons, notably Negroes, the pelvic muscles and fasciae are quite pliable and elastic, and little damage occurs during the birth of an infant. As a result, little or no relaxation can be detected even after many deliveries during which the patient has received no special medical care. Most women, however, are less fortunate. The tissues cannot stretch enough to permit the baby to pass easily, and, as a result, they give way. The end results of childbirth injuries depend upon how severe they were, how adequately they were repaired, and how completely they healed. That extensive damage can, for the most part, be prevented is suggested by the decrease in vaginal relaxation that has occurred as better obstetric care has become more generally available.

The most common injuries are those involving the lower vagina, the perineum, and the fasciae of the levator muscles. Multiple small tears around the urethra and clitoris may occur if the introitus is overstretched during delivery; these tears often bleed profusely. Superficial abrasions or deep tears may be noted in the vaginal mucosa. Such deep tears often cause severe bleeding and are prone to occur either in the vault of the vagina or over the spines. They often are produced during forceps rotation and extraction made necessary by abnormalities in pelvic architecture or by cephalopelvic disproportion, but they may also occur during less difficult operative extractions or even with spontaneous delivery.

Cervical lacerations that occur as a result of the effects of normal labor usually are shallow and bleed little. Those which are produced by the injudicious use of oxytocics or by attempts to deliver the infant before cer-

72

vical dilation is complete are likely to be more serious and may even extend upward into the lower uterine segment. Bleeding from the latter may be profuse, particularly if branches of the uterine artery are involved. The most serious of all the injuries is actual rupture of the uterine wall.

Only the injuries involving the perineum and external genitalia will be obvious to casual inspection. Those of the vagina, cervix, and uterus can be detected only by exposing the structures or by palpating the interior of the uterine cavity. Cervical lacerations usually bleed little and produce no immediate problem, but unless they are repaired, the abnormal cervix may subsequently require treatment. Also, the presence of vaginal tears may not be suspected. However, even though they do not bleed, they may become infected and serve as a source for entry of pathogenic bacteria. This danger can be reduced if they are sutured. In order to diagnose and correct these abnormalities, the cervix and vagina should be inspected after each delivery, and any defects that are observed should be repaired.

Plates 12 and 13

Episiotomy

Injury to the levators and the muscles and fasciae of the lower pelvis can be reduced to a minimum by episiotomy. Although episiotomy protects the posterior wall structures primarily, it also helps to minimize injury to the neck of the bladder and urethra by eliminating the resistance of the perineal structures that forces the presenting part forward to a position in which it compresses the neck of the bladder against the posterior surface of the pubis and pushes the soft tissue structures downward ahead of it as it descends during each contraction.

Episiotomy should be performed in almost all primigravidas and in any multipara whose fascial supports are well maintained. If the incision is made at the proper time, is accurately repaired, and heals well, it usually will be necessary to repeat the operation in each successive pregnancy.

Some kind of anesthetic is necessary before the perineum is incised, and whatever is selected for the delivery usually is adequate. Inhalation technics, local infiltration or pudendal block, saddle block, and other nerve root blocks all are satisfactory. The same anesthetic can be continued during the repair.

Plate 12

Mediolateral episiotomy

A. Episiotomy should usually be performed when the perineum is bulging well and when about 4 cm. of the fetal scalp is visible during a contraction. If the incision is made at this time, it will offer maximum protection to the tissues; if one waits until the perineum is completely thinned out, blanched, and ready to tear, much damage has already occurred and the end result will probably be less favorable.

B. The incision is made from the midline at the posterior fourchette toward the ischial tuberosity. The operator's two fingers in the vagina separate the labia and exert outward pressure on the perineum to flatten it slightly. No attempt is made to "iron out" the perineum. The incision must be deep enough to remove all perineal resistance to delivery of the infant; the fat in the ischiorectal fossa is usually exposed in an episiotomy of adequate depth. The repair is started only after the placenta has been expressed, the uterus is firmly contracted, and the cervix and vagina have been inspected for injury. This will prevent excessive blood loss from the uterus while the perineum is being repaired. In addition, if manual exploration of the uterus is necessary, either to remove the placenta or because of atony and bleeding, it cannot be done without removing the sutures if the incision has been adequately closed. Chromic 000 catgut on a round-point needle can be used to suture the incision.

C. The vaginal mucosa is repaired starting at the apex. Each bite should include the supporting tissues between the vagina and the rectum as well as the vaginal mucosa to provide stronger support. These sutures, which may be either interrupted or continuous, are carried past the cut edges of the hymen to the introitus.

D. The vaginal repair has been completed, and the levator muscle and its severed fascia are being approximated with interrupted sutures. The fascia on the medial side usually retracts somewhat toward the midline and beneath the more superficial structures, and it lies close to the anterior rectal wall, through which a suture can easily be placed. It is not necessary to use large sweeping bites to approximate these structures, and three or four sutures usually are adequate.

74

Plate 12

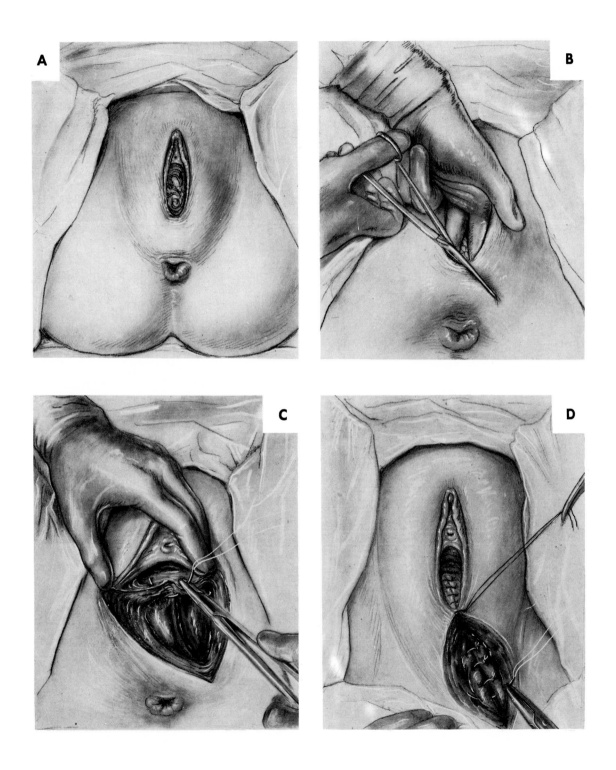

Plate 12 *Concluded*

Mediolateral episiotomy

E. The cut ends of the bulbocavernosus muscle are approximated as the first step in closing the more superficial layers of tissue. Since the muscle ends tend to retract upward, the skin edges must be pulled laterally and superiorly and a fairly deep bite taken to include the necessary structures. This is an important stitch; unless the tissues are properly approximated, the introitus will gape.

F. The muscle and fascial components of the urogenital diaphragm are approximated with interrupted sutures that are placed just beneath the skin.

G. The skin edges are approximated with a subcuticular catgut suture starting at the inferior end of the incision. This suture can be tied to one of the long ends of the mucosal stitch at the introitus.

H. The skin edges can also be approximated without sutures by applying Allis clamps, which are left in place for about thirty minutes. The results are comparable to those when sutures are placed.

Plate 12 *Concluded*

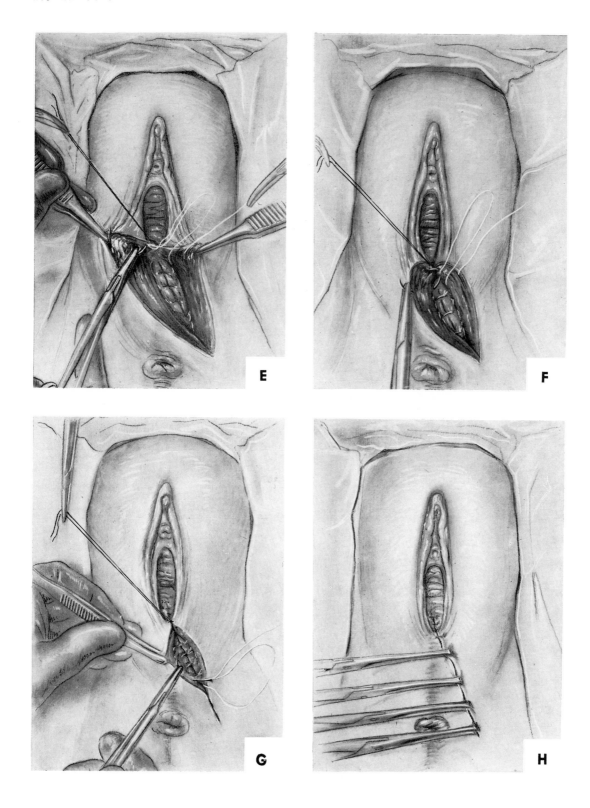

Plate 13

Median episiotomy

Many authorities prefer median to mediolateral episiotomy because it is easier to repair and more comfortable during the healing phase. The main disadvantages of the median type are the high incidence of sphincter and rectal tears and the possibility that the anterior rectal wall will be cut with the tips of the scissors. Although these can also occur with mediolateral episiotomy, they do so less frequently.

A. The perineum is incised from the midline of the posterior fourchette toward the anus until the anterior fibers of the anal sphincter can be recognized. The incision is made when the presenting part bulges the perineum well, as was described for mediolateral episiotomy.

B. The vaginal mucosa has been approximated with chromic 000 suture, and the separated bundles of the levator are being approximated anterior to the rectum with interrupted sutures. Three or four sutures are usually enough.

C. The cut ends of the bulbocavernosus muscle have been approximated and the urogenital diaphragm is now reconstructed. The cut edges of the muscle and fascia making up this structure are closed with interrupted stitches.

D. The skin is closed with a subcuticular chromic 000 suture, or Allis clamps can be used as previously described.

Plate 13

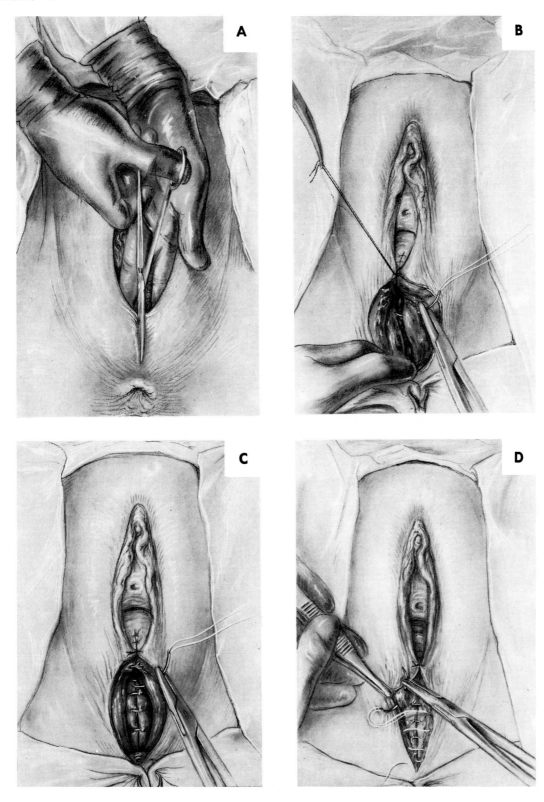

Plate 14

Repair of perineal injury

Injuries involving the perineal structures and the external genitalia usually are obvious, and all, except slight mucous membrane defects, should be repaired.

Tears involving the perineum may be superficial, extending down only as far as the muscle layer *(first-degree laceration)*, in which event the damage to the major supports is minimal, or they may be deeper and more disrupting. A *second-degree laceration* involves the urogenital diaphragm and levator structures, and in a *third-degree laceration* the anal sphincter is separated. A *fourth-degree laceration* involves the anterior rectal wall. Lacerations that are short and superficial usually occur in the midline, but if they extend upward into the vagina, they almost always involve one or both vaginal sulci. Lacerations, like episiotomies, are best repaired with chromic 000 catgut.

Perineal lacerations often occur during precipitate delivery before an anesthetic has been given or when only a minimal amount has been inhaled. Local infiltration or pudendal block is usually quite adequate for the subsequent repair and will obviate the need for inducing inhalation anesthesia.

A. A third-degree laceration. The sphincter, urogenital diaphragm, and levator fascia have been torn, and the laceration extends up each vaginal sulcus. In multiparas a better repair can often be obtained by dissecting the vaginal mucosa free from the posterior wall structures before the levators are approximated.

B. The levator bundles are approximated in the midline with interrupted sutures.

C. The mucosal extensions of the tear and the underlying supporting tissues have been closed, and the torn ends of the bulbocavernosus muscle are now approximated to aid in restoring a functional introitus.

D. The torn ends of the sphincter are pulled upward with forceps and approximated with a single interrupted suture.

E. Another catgut suture is placed in the sphincter at a right angle to the first one. These two stitches usually maintain adequate approximation until the tissues are healed.

F. The superficial muscle, fascial layers, and skin are then closed. No special aftercare is necessary except that mineral oil is ordered daily to keep the stools soft. The patient may be on a general diet, and it is not necessary to prescribe antibiotics.

Plate 14

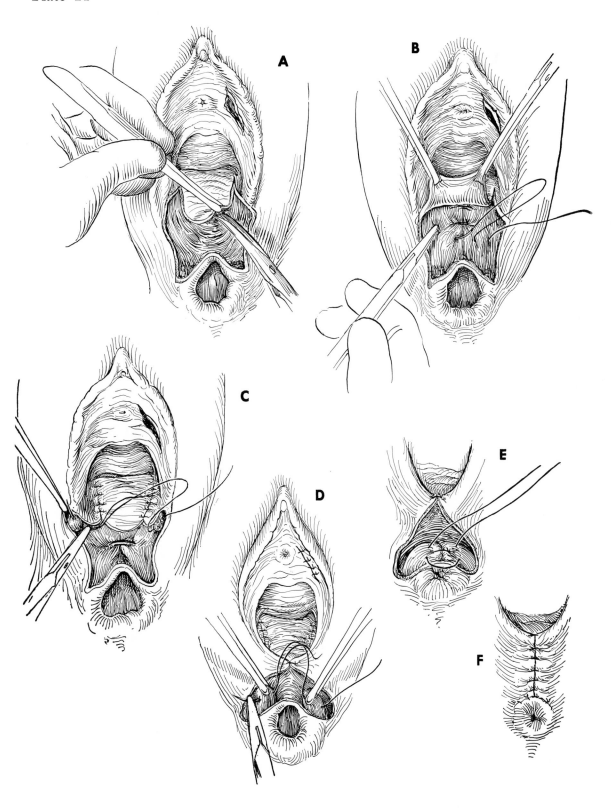

Plate 15

Cervical and vaginal lacerations

The cervix and vagina often are injured during delivery, and the lacerations are not usually obvious because they are hidden within the vagina and because those of the cervix usually bleed little. The only method by which such injuries can be detected is inspection of the lower birth canal after each delivery.

A. Right-angle retractors are inserted anteriorly and posteriorly, and the cervix is grasped with ring forceps and its entire circumference inspected. If the physician responsible for the delivery does not have a sterile assistant, the circulating nurse can hold the anterior retractor in place by grasping the handle through a sterile towel.

B. The vault of the vagina posteriorly and the lateral fornices are now exposed by manipulating the cervix with the sponge forceps. Lacerations that are hidden behind the redundant dilated cervix are thereby exposed to view.

C. Cervical lacerations more than 1 cm. long should be repaired even though they are not bleeding. The raw edges are approximated with interrupted sutures of chromic 000 catgut, each stitch being placed through the entire thickness of the cervix. The apex of a deep laceration may not be obvious if it is above the vaginal vault. Unless the highest suture can be placed accurately above the upper end of the tear, a laparotomy is justifiable because extensive bleeding can occur from an unligated vessel.

D. Vaginal lacerations are also repaired with chromic 000 catgut. Bleeding is usually far more profuse than from tears in the cervix, and a continuous lock stitch often provides better hemostasis. A fine atraumatic needle produces less bleeding than a large one through which the suture material is looped. It usually is not necessary to insert a pack unless hemostasis is incomplete, in which event the vagina is packed tightly with gauze, which is left in place about twelve hours.

Occasionally bleeding from vaginal lacerations is so profuse that neither an accurate appraisal nor an adequate repair is possible. In such instances, or when lack of assistance makes exposure of the injured tissue impossible, the vagina can be tightly packed as a temporary expedient. This will control bleeding until the repair can be made subsequently under more favorable circumstances.

Adequate anesthesia is essential for repair of vaginal lacerations. Pudendal block may be sufficient for the exposure and suture of injuries in the lower vagina, but usually it is inadequate for injuries that extend to the vault.

82

Plate 15

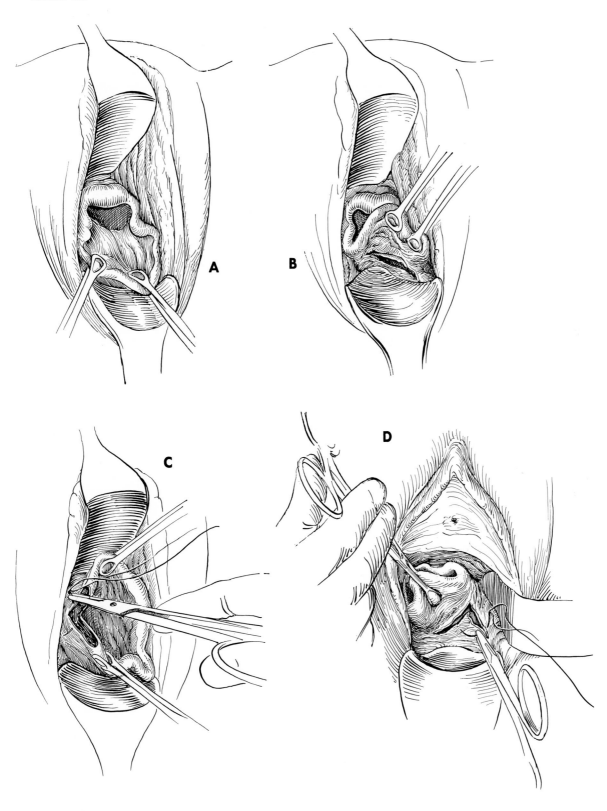

Plate 16

Repair of old cervical lacerations

Lacerations of the cervix that were sustained during a previous delivery but that either were not sutured at the time or failed to heal can be repaired at subsequent delivery. If proper healing occurs, the condition of the cervix will be much improved after involution is complete.

A. The already healed and epithelized edges of the laceration must be excised to permit approximation of raw tissue for optimum healing. The cervix is grasped with ring forceps on either side of the old defect, and a V-shaped portion of tissue is excised from the rim of the cervix to the apex of the tear.

B. The defect is closed with interrupted sutures of chromic 000 catgut. At least partial healing almost always occurs.

Plate 16

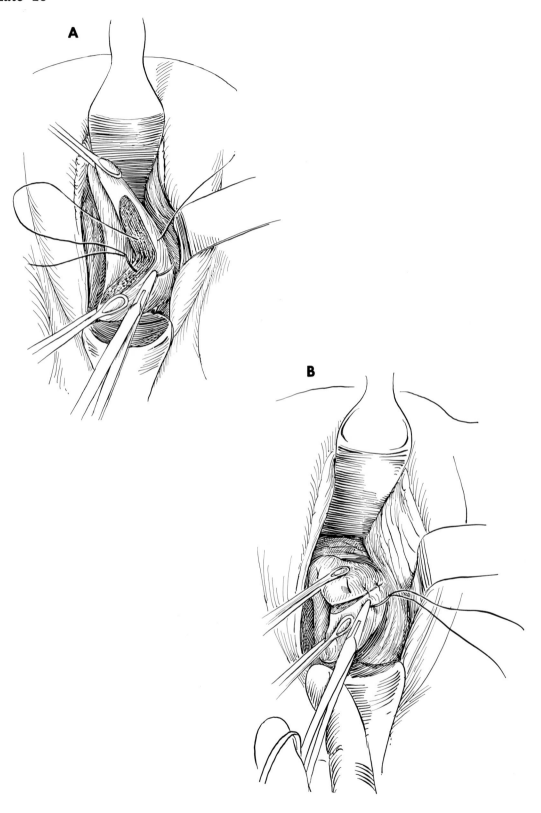

Chapter 7

Forceps delivery

Several hundred different types of obstetric forceps have been devised, but all the effective ones are variants of the prototype of the modern instrument that was developed and used so successfully by the Chamberlens during the seventeenth century. The principal purpose of obstetric forceps is to *extract* the head from the birth canal or to *rotate* it to a position more favorable for delivery. Rotation almost always is followed immediately by extraction. A certain amount of compression of the fetal head must of necessity occur to permit traction, but the instrument is never used either as a means of decreasing the size of the skull or to dilate the cervix.

INDICATIONS

The major indication for the use of forceps is *cessation of progress* during the second stage of labor as a result of inadequate uterine contractions, malposition of the fetus, or abnormal configuration of the birth canal. Forceps delivery may be considered, unless some other method of termination will be safer for the mother and her baby, if the head fails to descend or a transverse or posterior position remains unchanged during a two-hour period in the second stage of labor in spite of what seem to be effective contractions, or if progress ceases because of inadequate contractions that cannot be corrected by the judicious use of oxytocin. Occasionally the head descends to the pelvic floor but fails to advance farther because of a combination of factors, such as poor contractions, inability to make effective use of the secondary powers, and soft tissue resistance. If the baby has not been expelled within an hour, extraction is warranted.

Forceps delivery may prevent death from *intrauterine anoxia* during the second stage of labor if the signs of fetal distress are detected before irreparable damage has resulted from the reduced oxygenation of the infant's brain. It is well to count the fetal heart rate frequently and to administer oxygen to the mother whenever any unusual variation is detected.

An irregularity or decrease in rate, particularly if it slows more than 20 or 30 beats per minute or falls below 100 beats per minute, or the passage of meconium in vertex positions suggests that oxygenation is deficient. The expulsion of meconium in breech positions is less significant. Before applying forceps under these circumstances, the operator must be certain not only that delivery is necessary but that it can be accomplished readily, because forceful extraction from a high station or delivery through an undilated cervix may injure the baby as much as or more than will the reduced oxygen supply. It is also likely to damage the mother's soft tissues extensively.

The expulsive efforts usually necessary to complete the second stage of labor are undesirable for women with *heart disease, pulmonary tuberculosis or other respiratory lesions, and hypertension and other vascular lesions* and should be avoided whenever possible. Unless delivery can be anticipated with a few contractions, as is usual with multiparous women, the infant should be extracted soon after perineal distention is observed and before the patient begins to bear down involuntarily.

Elective or prophylactic low forceps delivery combined with episiotomy is often used as a means of shortening the perineal phase of labor. Many obstetricians choose this as a regular method for conducting delivery and, when properly performed, it adds nothing to the risk to either the mother or the infant. In fact, it permits the performance of episiotomy relatively early, before the tissues have been stretched and damaged by the emerging head. This operation is safe and effective as a regular procedure only when performed in the hospital by physicians who are trained in the use of forceps and who adhere rigidly to the requirements for low forceps delivery.

REQUIREMENTS

The use of forceps is contraindicated, even though there is need to deliver the infant, unless certain requirements can be met.

The cervix must be completely dilated and preferably retracted. Unless the cervix is fully dilated, it is almost certain to be lacerated, perhaps severely, during the attempts to apply the blades and extract the infant. It is possible to enlarge the opening enough to permit delivery by incising the cervix if it is thin and already dilated 7 to 8 cm., but attempts at manual dilation usually tear the tissue rather than stretch it.

The head must be presenting in a position that will permit delivery, and it must be engaged. The deeper the head has descended into the birth canal, the less the trauma from forceps delivery. The operator must make certain by vaginal examination and, if necessary, by x-ray study that the biparietal diameter has actually passed through the inlet. A large caput or the lowest portion of a greatly elongated skull may be felt well below the spines, giving a false impression of the true state of affairs.

√ *There must be no serious bony or soft tissue obstruction.* Minor degrees of pelvic contraction do not necessarily contraindicate forceps delivery;
√ in fact, such contractions may serve as prime indications for the use of the forceps. However, serious disproportion and the presence of tumors that obstruct the birth canal usually do contraindicate forceps delivery.

√ *An anesthetic should be administered.* The manipulations that are necessary to apply the blades and to extract the infant are painful, and anesthesia is almost always required.

√ *The membranes must be ruptured, and the bladder should be emptied.*

√ *The operator must be familiar with the mechanism of normal labor and experienced in forceps delivery.* The fact that this requirement is mentioned last is no indication of its relative importance. The ability to select the appropriate time for forceps delivery, to apply the blades accurately, and to follow as closely as possible the normal mechanism of labor may be the difference between a successful termination and serious injury or even death of the infant.

Plate 17

Forceps—construction and application

Obstetric forceps consist of two halves, each of which is made up of a *blade* designed to fit the infant's head, a *shank* that connects the blade to the handle, a *lock* that permits articulation of the halves of the instrument, and a *handle* from which traction is applied. The right half of the forceps is held in the operator's right hand while the blade is applied to the right side of the maternal pelvis, and the left half is held in the left hand and applied to the left side of the birth canal. The blades are designed to grasp the head firmly enough to permit extraction with a minimum of compression and to follow the curve of the birth canal. All edges are smooth and rounded to reduce the possibility of cutting the soft tissues. Open blades are preferable for traction because the scalp tissues bulge through the fenestra when the forceps are locked, thus preventing slipping. Rotation of the head can be more easily accomplished with smooth, solid blade instruments if the pelvis is small, but for most operations the open blades are satisfactory.

Although most forceps are similar in form, minor variations may make some instruments a little better for certain specific maneuvers. In general, however, a physician can perform almost any forceps operation quite adequately if he familiarizes himself with the use of forceps of the Simpson type, Kielland forceps, and one such as the Piper forceps for extraction of the aftercoming head.

Plate 17 continued on p. 90.

Plate 17 *Continued*

Forceps—construction and application

A. Pelvic curve—When the forceps are placed on a tabletop, the superior surfaces of the blades curve smoothly upward, the tips being 7.5 to 8 cm. about the level of the table. This permits the blades to follow the curve of the birth canal, thereby minimizing soft tissue damage when they are applied properly.

B. Cephalic curve—The widest diameter of the cephalic curve is usually about 7.5 cm. Thus, when the forceps are properly applied, the cephalic curve is only slightly smaller in diameter than the head it is intended to grasp. The cephalic curve of the Simpson type of forceps is relatively long and tapered, which facilitates application when the head is molded and elongated without reducing its general usefulness.

The shank varies in length, and an instrument with a long shank should be selected for midforceps delivery. The DeLee modification of the Simpson forceps is quite satisfactory for this operation.

Most of the forceps used in this country are equipped with an English type of lock that permits easy and stable articulation. The forceps can be locked only when the shank of the right half of the instrument lies above the shank of the left half.

C. The term *cephalic application* of forceps indicates that the blades have been applied in the occipitomental diameter of the head. This is the ideal application and may be possible regardless of the position of the head within the pelvis.

With *pelvic application,* the blades lie in the pelvis, with their superior surfaces directed toward the pubis and the pelvic curve, corresponding to the curve of the birth canal, as shown in *A.* For direct occiput anterior and direct occiput posterior positions, the blades are also in cephalic application, but if the head has not yet completely rotated, the forceps may grasp the head in an undesirable manner; for example, one blade may be applied to the face and the other to the occiput. The possibility of injuring the baby is increased.

The *position* of the forceps in the pelvis is indicated by the direction of the plane that passes at right angles through the blades. For instance, if each blade lies against the lateral pelvic wall, with the superior surface directed anteriorly, the forceps are in a transverse position. If one blade lies in the hollow of the sacrum and the other behind the pubis, the position is anteroposterior. If the left blade lies in the left anterior quadrant and the right blade lies in the right posterior quadrant of the pelvis, the forceps are in the right oblique position.

90

Plate 17

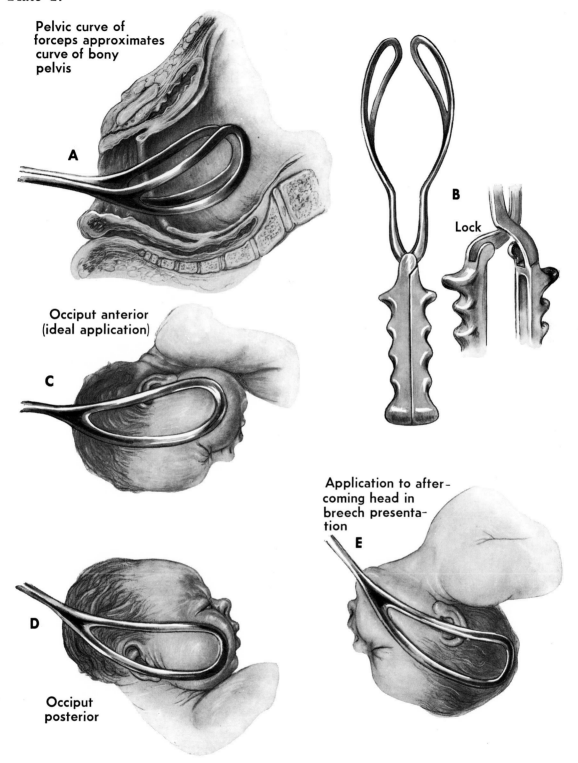

Pelvic curve of forceps approximates curve of bony pelvis

A

B

Lock

Occiput anterior (ideal application)

C

Application to after-coming head in breech presenta-tion

E

D

Occiput posterior

D. Forceps application in occiput posterior positions. The head usually is elongated, and an instrument with a long cephalic curve is to be preferred.

E. Forceps application for delivery of the aftercoming head and in face positions.

Plate 18

Types of forceps delivery

As a general rule, forceps delivery becomes easier and less damaging in the more advanced stages of labor. If the cervix is completely dilated and retracted and the head has descended to the pelvic floor and has rotated to an anterior position, the infant can usually be extracted easily and safely. This is not necessarily true of midforceps deliveries. Before a decision is made to terminate labor by forceps extraction, the physician must make certain by vaginal and, when indicated, by x-ray examination that the size and shape of the pelvis are adequate for delivery, that the cervix is completely dilated, and that engagement has occurred. X-ray studies are particularly important in determining whether the biparietal diameter of the head has passed the pelvic inlet.

A. Classification of forceps deliveries according to areas in the pelvis.

B. *Floating and high forceps deliveries* can almost never be performed safely. In the former, the head lies free above the plane of the inlet and can barely be reached. In the latter, the head is entering the pelvis, usually in a transverse position, but its lowest portion has not yet descended to the level of the ischial spines. The head is unengaged because the biparietal diameter is above the inlet.

C. In *high midforceps deliveries*, the biparietal diameter of the head has passed through the inlet, and the lowest portion lies between the level of the ischial spines and the perineal floor. The head usually is partially flexed, and the occiput has begun to rotate toward the anterior quadrant of the pelvis, although it often is still in a transverse or even a posterior position.

D. In *low midforceps deliveries*, the head has descended beyond the perineal floor and usually is fairly well flexed and rotated anteriorly, although it may still be in a transverse or posterior position.

E. In *low forceps deliveries* the scalp is visible through the distended introitus during a contraction, and the sagittal suture occupies the anteroposterior diameter of the outlet, with the posterior fontanel beneath the pubic arch.

Plate 18

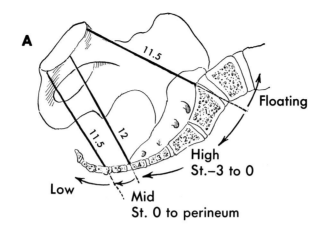

A

11.5

12

11.5

Floating

High
St. –3 to 0

Low

Mid
St. 0 to perineum

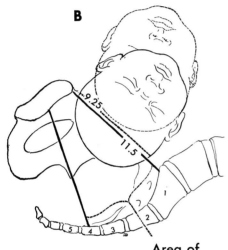

B

9.25

11.5

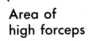

Area of
high forceps

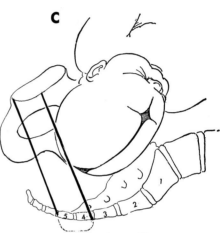

C

Area of high midforceps

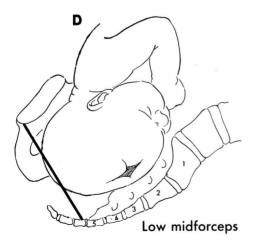

D

Low midforceps

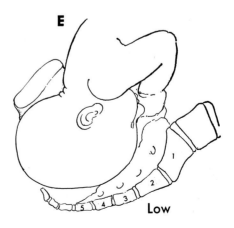

E

Low

93

Plate 19

Low forceps delivery

Low forceps delivery is performed after the head has rotated to an anterior position and is visible at the introitus during a contraction. Low forceps delivery may become necessary because the patient is unable or unwilling to bear down and the force of the primary powers alone is inadequate to complete the delivery. However, it is more often an elective procedure. As soon as the head is crowning well, but before the perineal structures have been overstretched or torn, the perineum is incised and the head is lifted over the perineum. When properly performed, this procedure adds nothing to the risk; on the contrary, it tends to decrease soft tissue damage.

Anesthesia is usually necessary. The delivery and subsequent repair can be performed with pudendal block, caudal block, low spinal, or inhalation technics.

A. With the patient in lithotomy position and under anesthesia, the position of the infant is determined by vaginal palpation. The forceps will be applied in ideal cephalic application, with the pelvic curve of the instrument corresponding to the curve of the birth canal (transverse position). Episiotomy is performed at this time.

B. The handle of the left blade of the forceps is grasped between the thumb and the first two fingers of the operator's left hand and held over the mother's right groin, with the tip of the blade through the introitus between the left frontal portion of the head and the first two fingers of the operator's right hand, over which it will pass into the vagina. The blade is steadied and guided by the thumb. The fingers need not be introduced deeply because the cervix has retracted upward, and there is no chance of impinging it between the tip of the forceps and the skull.

C. The position of the forceps blade in the pelvic outlet.

94

Plate 19

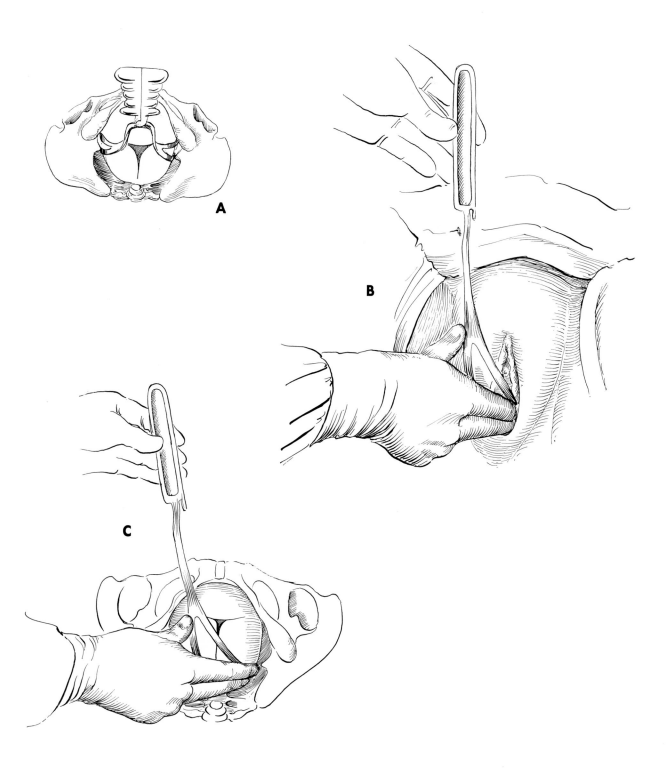

Plate 19 *Continued*

Low forceps delivery

D. The blade is introduced by simultaneously depressing the handle and swinging it toward the midline as the blade is pushed over the first two fingers of the operator's right hand into the vagina. This maneuver permits the concave inner surface of the blade to glide around the convex fetal head while the pelvic curve adapts itself to the curving birth canal. Little force is required to introduce the blade, but its application may be facilitated by pouring a small amount of green soap over the palmar surface of the right hand as the fingers are inserted through the introitus.

E. The same maneuver in lateral view. After the blade is introduced, it is in ideal application. An assistant holds the left blade in position while the right one is applied by the operator.

Plate 19 *Continued*

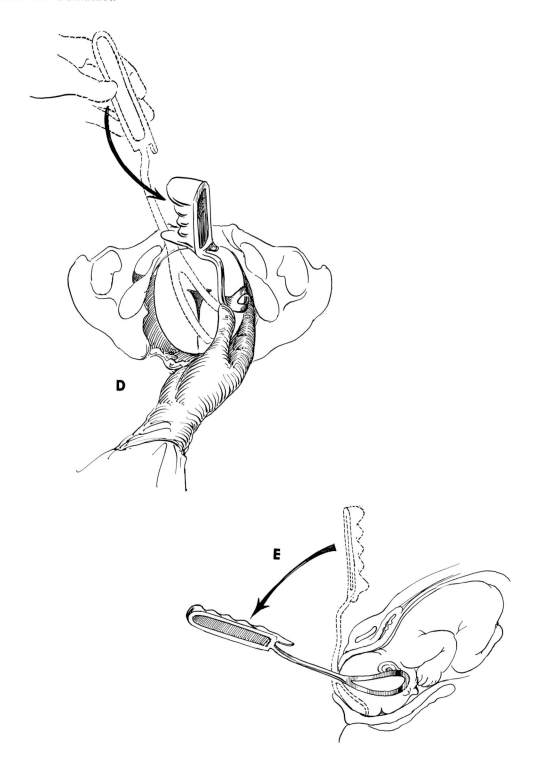

Plate 19 *Continued*

Low forceps delivery

F. The first two fingers of the left hand are introduced through the introitus into the right side of the pelvis, and the handle of the right half of the instrument held in the operator's right hand is suspended over the patient's left groin.

G. The right blade is introduced by a maneuver similar to that by which the left blade was applied. The shank of the right blade now overlies the shank of the left blade, and the forceps can be articulated by closing the handles. If the blades are properly applied, it should be possible to lock the forceps without difficulty. If the handles cannot be closed easily, the forceps may not be accurately placed because the position may not have been diagnosed accurately; consequently, it should be rechecked before continuing the procedure.

H. Before the operator attempts to extract the head, he should make certain that he has achieved a satisfactory application by locating the posterior fontanel and palpating the sagittal and occipital sutures.

Plate 19 *Continued*

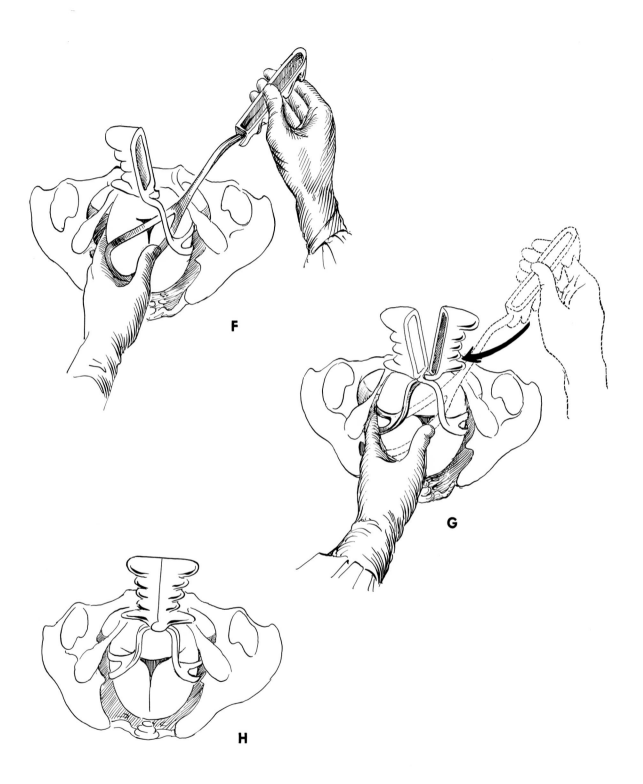

F

G

H

Plate 19 *Continued*

Low forceps delivery

I. The operator seats himself comfortably on a stool in front of the patient and grasps the forceps firmly with both hands. The most effective force at this stage is obtained by a combination of outward and downward traction (Pajot's maneuver). The downward force is obtained by firm pressure on the superior surface of the shank of the instrument with the fingers of the right hand and by upward pressure on the inferior surface of the handle with the thumbs. When this pressure is combined with outward traction, the occiput is brought down beneath the symphysis while the anterior portion of the head is emerging over the perineum.

J. The slightly elongated head is now brought through the introitus, following the plane of the outlet, by a combination of traction and upward pressure with both thumbs. This extends the head as it is pulled downward and mimics the normal mechanism. If the head is extended too soon or is extended without being extracted simultaneously, the long cephalic diameters that are forced through the introitus will distend the perineal structures and perhaps damage the soft tissues unnecessarily.

Plate 19 *Continued*

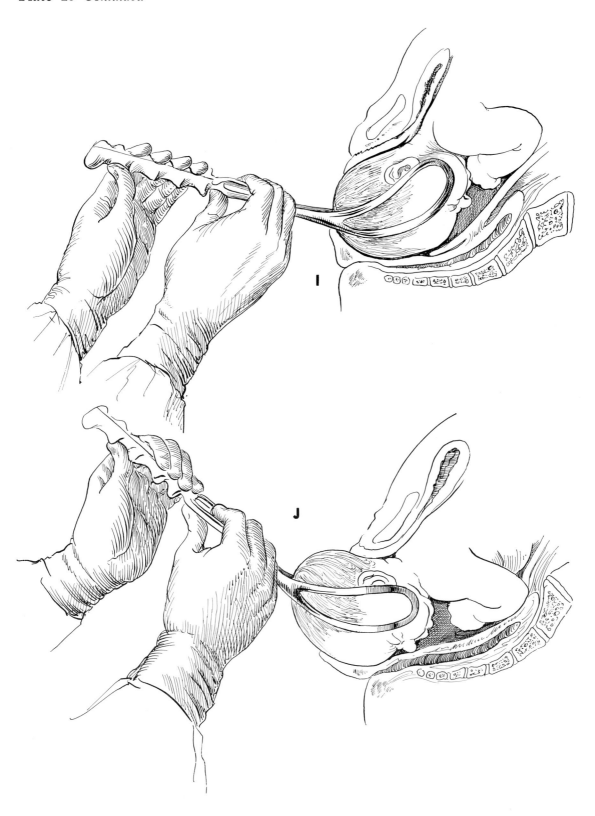

Plate 19 *Concluded*

Low forceps delivery

K. With further traction and extension, the forehead appears over the introitus.

L. At this stage, it may be wise to remove the forceps, thereby decreasing slightly the diameters of the head as it emerges. The forceps are disarticulated, and the blades are removed by a process exactly the reverse of that by which they were applied. The handle of the right blade is raised toward the left groin, thereby rotating the cephalic curve around the head. The left blade is removed in a similar manner. The delivery of the head is then completed by upward pressure on the forehead or by sweeping the chin out by inserting the fingers into the vagina beneath it and applying gentle traction.

Plate 19 *Concluded*

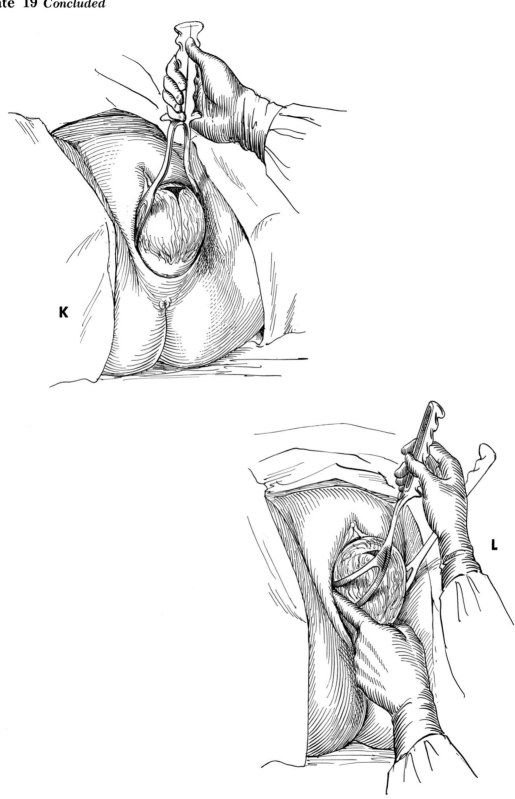

Plate 20

Low midforceps delivery—occiput anterior position

The maneuvers for performing low midforceps delivery in occiput anterior position are similar to those for low forceps delivery, but slight modifications are necessary because the head is at a higher station in the birth canal.

A. After the operator has diagnosed the position with certainty, he inserts four, instead of two, fingers of the right hand into the vagina between the lateral pelvic wall and the infant's head. The left blade of the forceps is introduced into the vagina in a manner similar to that described for low forceps delivery.

B. Deeper insertion of the guiding fingers is necessary not only because the head is higher but because occasionally the cervix has not yet retracted completely and may be caught between the tips of the forceps and the infant's head. This can be prevented by passing the fingers inside the cervix so that the blade, when introduced between the palmar surfaces of the fingers and the infant's skull, will certainly be within the cervical opening. Cervical laceration is more likely to occur if retraction is incomplete, even though the blades are properly applied.

C. After applying the right blade and checking to make certain that the forceps have been applied within the cervical opening and in ideal application, the handles are grasped in the manner described for low forceps delivery and the traction force is applied by Pajot's maneuver.

D. After the head appears at the introitus, the remainder of the delivery is essentially that of low forceps extraction.

Plate 20

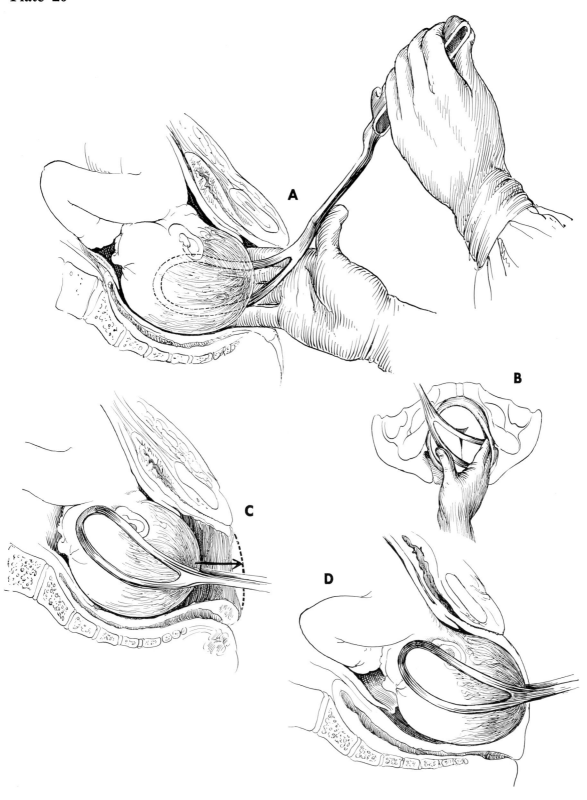

Plate 21

Forceps delivery–occiput right anterior position

It sometimes is necessary to extract the infant with forceps before complete anterior rotation of the occiput has occurred. If the head has descended deeply into the pelvis and has begun to distend the pelvic floor, there is no particular risk involved, but delivery may be difficult and traumatic if the presenting part is higher, even though engagement has occurred. Until the head reaches the pelvic floor, flexion is usually incomplete unless the pelvic capacity is reduced, in which event the head must flex completely in order to descend.

The necessary manipulations can often be carried out under pudendal nerve block anesthesia if the head lies deep in the birth canal, but saddle block or inhalation anesthesia is usually preferable for midforceps delivery. Episiotomy is desirable for almost all primigravidas and for many multiparas and is best performed before the blades are applied. Although this does increase the blood loss slightly, it reduces soft tissue damage.

A. The desired application. The sagittal suture parallels the left oblique diameter of the pelvis, with the posterior fontanel directed toward the right anterior quadrant and the anterior fontanel directed toward the left posterior quadrant. The blades are in ideal cephalic application in the right oblique diameter of the pelvis.

B. After the position has been accurately determined, the operator inserts all four fingers of the right hand into the vagina between the infant's head and the lateral pelvic wall. The handle of the left half of the forceps is held in the operator's left hand, and the tip of the blade is inserted through the introitus between the palmar surfaces of the fingers and the left side of the infant's forehead.

C. As the forceps handle is swung downward and toward the patient's left thigh, the blade slides around the head and into the vagina, where it lies between the left side of the infant's face and the lateral pelvic wall slightly anterior to the ischial spine.

D. The forceps blade is adjusted into position by manipulating the handle with the left hand and the blade with the fingertips of the right hand and the ball of the thumb. No attempt is made at this time to apply the blade in ideal position on the head.

Plate 21

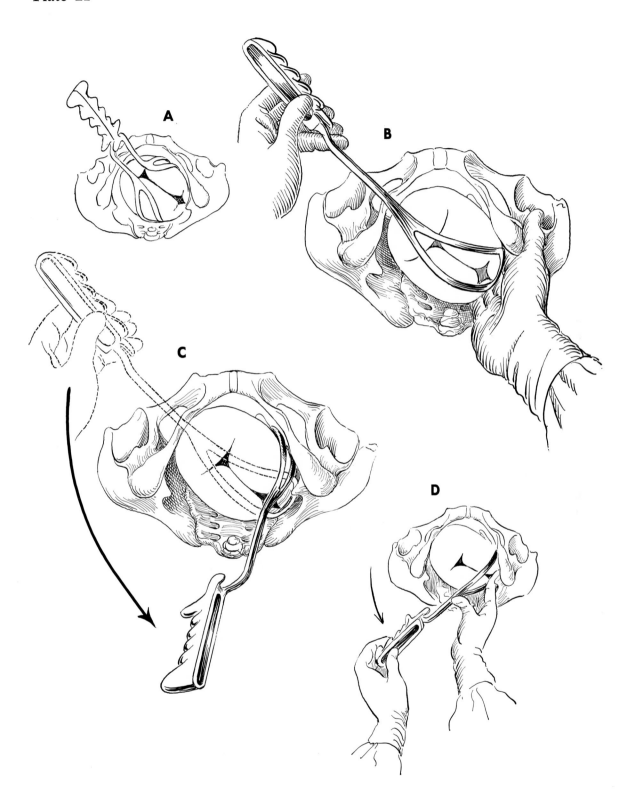

A

B

C

D

Plate **21** *Continued*

Forceps delivery—occiput right anterior position

E. While an assistant holds the left half of the instrument in place in the left side of the pelvis, the right blade is introduced by the operator. The four fingers of the operator's left hand are inserted into the right posterior quadrant of the pelvis, and the tip of the blade is introduced between the fingers and the right parietal eminence of the fetal head.

F. As the handle is swung downward and toward the mother's right thigh, the blade slides around the head and into the pelvis, coming to rest in ideal application in the occipitomental diameter over the right side of the fetal head.

Plate 21 *Continued*

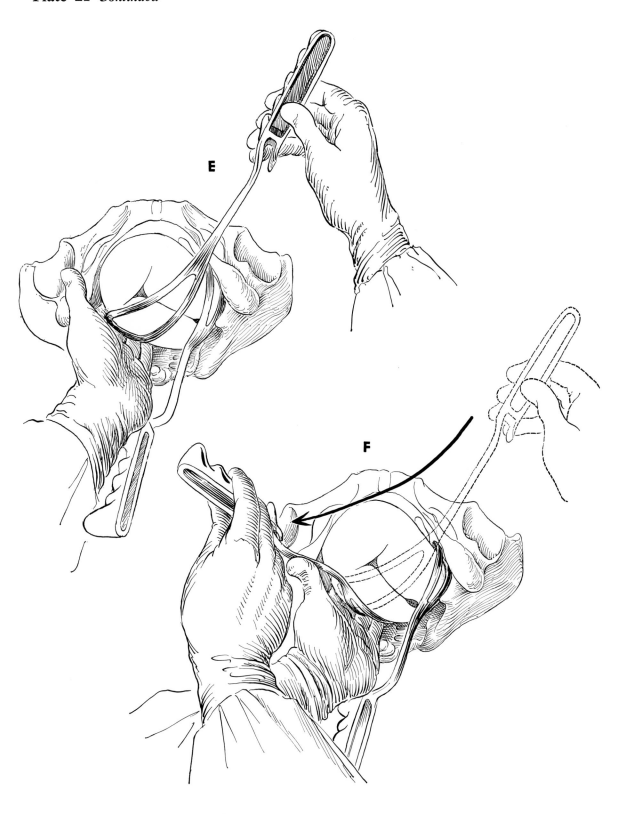

E

F

Plate 21 *Concluded*

Forceps delivery—occiput right anterior position

G. Since the right blade lies in proper cephalic application in the right oblique diameter of the pelvis and the left blade in pelvic, but not in cephalic, application in the left lateral pelvis, it will be impossible to articulate the forceps. The left blade is manipulated around the head toward the anterior pelvis with the fingers and the thumb of the operator's right hand until it lies in the right oblique diameter of the pelvis and in the occipitomental diameter of the left side of the head, with its shank beneath the shank of the right blade.

H. The forceps can now be articulated, after which the operator reexamines the patient to make certain that the blades have been applied properly. Slight adjustments can be made by partially disarticulating the instrument and manipulating the blades into a more satisfactory position with the fingertips while the other hand steadies the handle.

Using the modified Pajot's maneuver, traction is applied approximately in the axis of the birth canal. It usually is not necessary to make a definite effort to rotate the head if the pelvic architecture is normal; as it descends with traction, it will rotate spontaneously until the occipital portion lies beneath the symphysis, from which it can easily be extracted.

Plate 21 *Concluded*

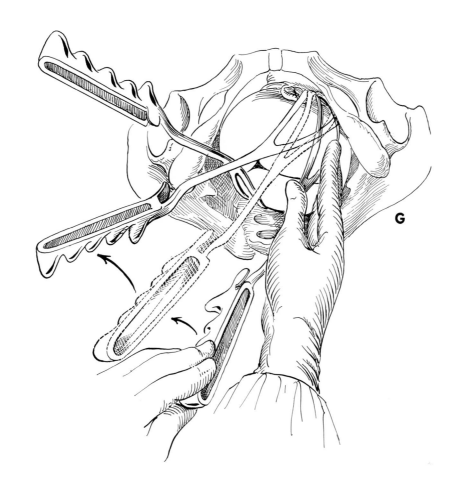

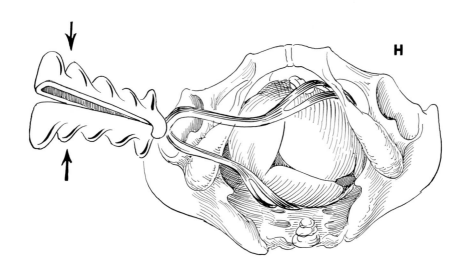

Plate 22

Forceps delivery—occiput left anterior position

A. The desired application. The sagittal suture parallels the right oblique diameter of the pelvis, with the posterior fontanel directed toward the left anterior quadrant and the anterior fontanel directed toward the right posterior quadrant. The blades are in ideal application in the left oblique diameter of the pelvis.

B. After the position has been accurately determined, all four fingers of the right hand are inserted into the vagina between the left parietal bone and the posterolateral pelvic wall. The handle of the left half of the forceps is held in the operator's left hand, and the tip of the blade is inserted through the introitus between the palmar surfaces of his fingers and the left side of the infant's head. As the handle of the forceps is swung downward and toward the patient's left thigh, the blade slides around the infant's head and into the left posterior quadrant of the vagina, where it lies over the left side of the head, approximately but not quite in the occipitomental diameter.

Plate 22

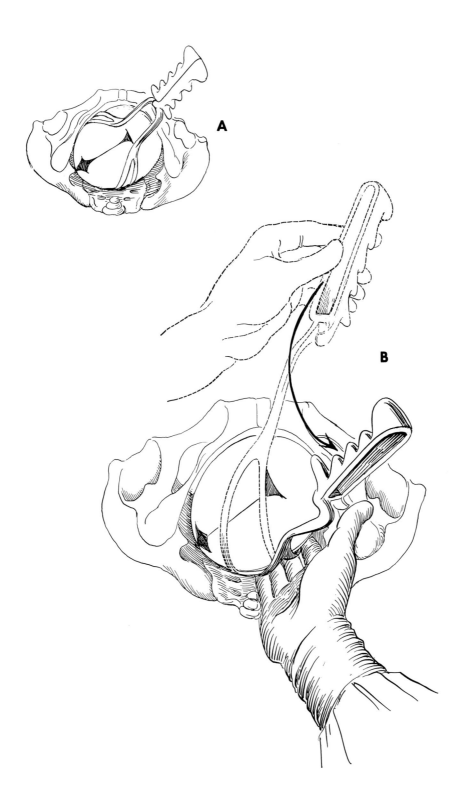

A

B

Plate 22 *Continued*

Forceps delivery—occiput left anterior position

C. The four fingers of the left hand are inserted between the anterior portion of the right parietal bone and the right lateral pelvic wall. The handle of the right half of the instrument is held in the operator's right hand over the patient's left groin, with the tip of the blade between the operator's fingers and the infant's skull.

D. As the handle is depressed and swung toward the patient's right thigh, the blade slides around the infant's head and into the right side of the pelvis, where it comes to rest over the anterior portion of the right parietal bone. Since the left blade lies in the left oblique diameter of the pelvis, where the head can be grasped properly, it will be impossible to approximate the handles until the position of the right blade has been adjusted.

Plate 22 *Continued*

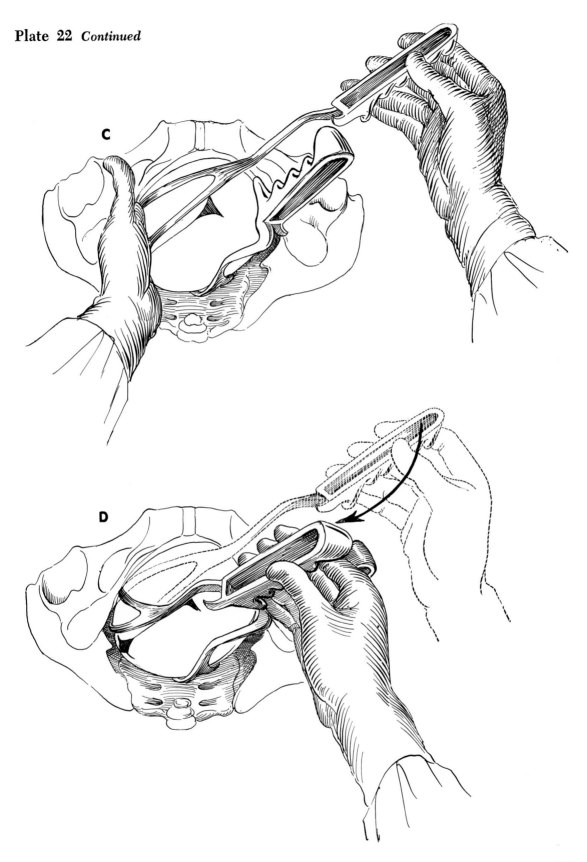

Plate 22 *Concluded*

Forceps delivery—occiput left anterior position

E. The right blade is manipulated anteriorly around the side of the infant's head until it lies in ideal cephalic application in the left oblique diameter of the pelvis.

F. The handle of the left half is now raised until it can be articulated with the right handle, thereby bringing the blade into proper position in the occipito-mental diameter of the head. After the application has been checked, the infant's head is extracted.

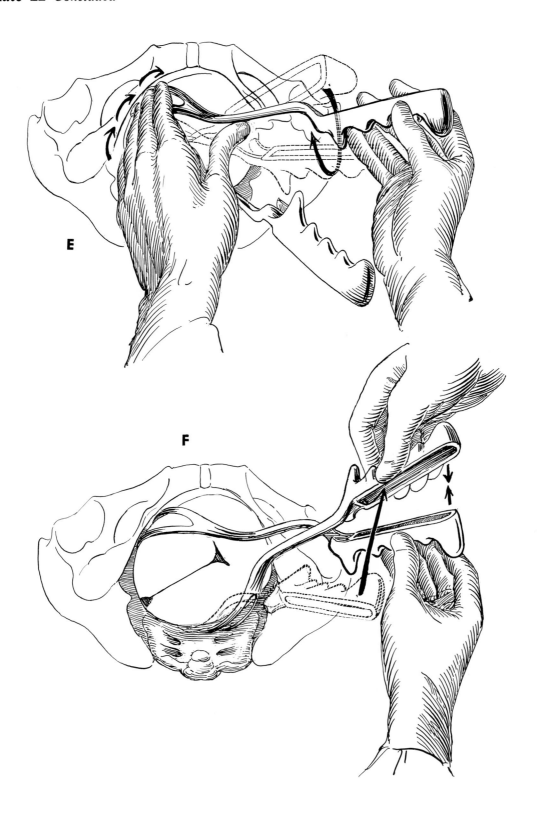

Plate 22 *Concluded*

E

F

Plates 23 and 24

Forceps delivery—occiput transverse positions

When it is necessary to deliver an infant from an occiput transverse position, the head is usually well above the pelvic floor and flexion is incomplete. Relatively profound anesthesia, such as that provided by saddle block or inhalation technics, usually is necessary to eliminate pain and to provide enough relaxation of the voluntary muscles to permit the necessary manipulations.

It may be difficult to apply forceps to the head in a transverse position, particularly if it is molded or elongated. Whenever possible, the head should be rotated manually to an anterior position, thereby facilitating the application of the blades and the subsequent extraction.

Plate 23

Forceps delivery—occiput left transverse position

A. The head is engaged, and the most dependent portion lies below the level of the ischial spines. The sagittal suture parallels the transverse diameter of the pelvis, with the posterior fontanel directed toward the left lateral pelvic wall and the anterior fontanel directed toward the right lateral pelvic wall and at a level only slightly above that of the former. There often is moderate molding and caput formation, which obscures the usual landmarks. In this event, position is diagnosed by passing the entire hand into the vagina until an ear can be identified.

B. The desired application. The blades are in ideal cephalic application in the anteroposterior diameter of the pelvis.

C. The four fingers of the right hand are introduced into the vagina between the left parietal bone and the sacrum. The handle of the left half of the instrument is held over the mother's left groin, with the tip of the blade through the introitus between the fingers and the infant's head.

118

Plate 23

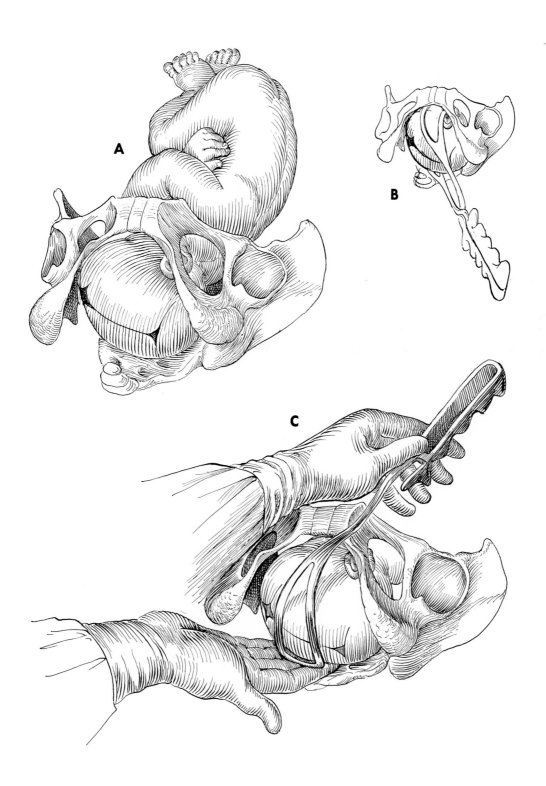

Plate 23 *Continued*

Forceps delivery—occiput left transverse position

D. As the handle is lowered and swung toward the mother's left thigh, the blade slides over the palmar surfaces of the operator's fingers and around the infant's head until it lies in the hollow of the sacrum and over the left parietal bone, with its anterior surface directed toward the left lateral pelvic wall. Unless the head has descended almost to the pelvic floor, it may not be possible to apply the blade in ideal cephalic application.

E. The four fingers of the left hand are inserted into the vagina between the infant's face and the right lateral pelvic wall. The handle of the right blade is held over the mother's left groin, with its tip inserted through the introitus between the fingers and the infant's head.

Plate 23 *Continued*

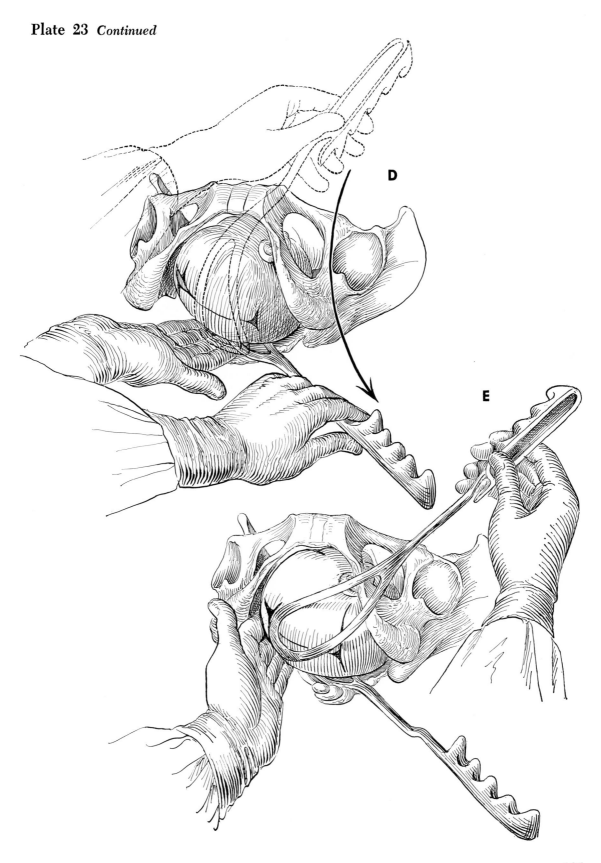

D

E

Plate **23** *Continued*

Forceps delivery—occiput left transverse position

F. As the handle is swung downward and toward the mother's right thigh, the blade slides between the operator's fingers and the fetal skull into the right side of the pelvis. It may lie between the face and the lateral pelvic wall, but it is more likely to be somewhat farther forward in the right anterior quadrant overlying the anterior portion of the right parietal bone and the infant's cheek.

Plate 23 *Continued*

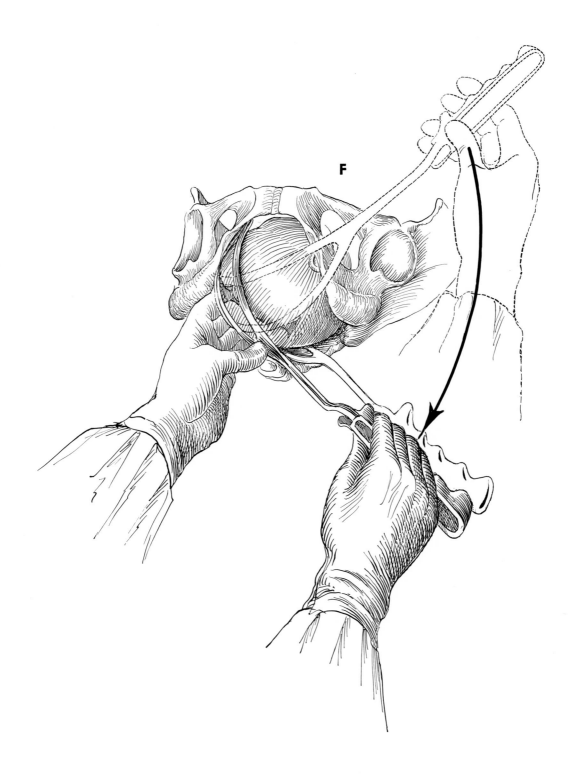

F

Plate 23 *Concluded*

Forceps delivery—occiput left transverse position

G. The right blade is manipulated over the cheek and around the infant's head by a seesaw motion, with the fingers and thumb of the operator's left hand on the blade and those of his right hand controlling the handle.

H. The right blade finally comes into position beneath the pubic arch parallel to the posterior blade, with the pelvic curve of the instrument directed toward the left side of the pelvis. The forceps should be close to the ideal cephalic application, particularly if the head is reasonably well flexed.

I. The handle of the right blade is passed above the handle of the left blade, and the forceps are articulated.

J. The final position of the blades in relationship to the landmarks on the head is checked after the forceps have been locked.

K. Although the head will usually rotate to an anterior position as it is pulled downward, sometimes it is necessary to turn it by rotating the handles of the forceps through a 90-degree arc from left to right until the posterior fontanel lies beneath the symphysis and the pelvic curve of the instrument approximates that of the birth canal. If the transverse position is a result of reduced anteroposterior pelvic diameters (platypellic or rachitic pelvis), it may not be possible to rotate the head until it has passed the promontory of the sacrum. Under these conditions the head is pulled downward in the transverse diameter until it can be turned as it is extracted through the outlet.

124

Plate 23 *Concluded*

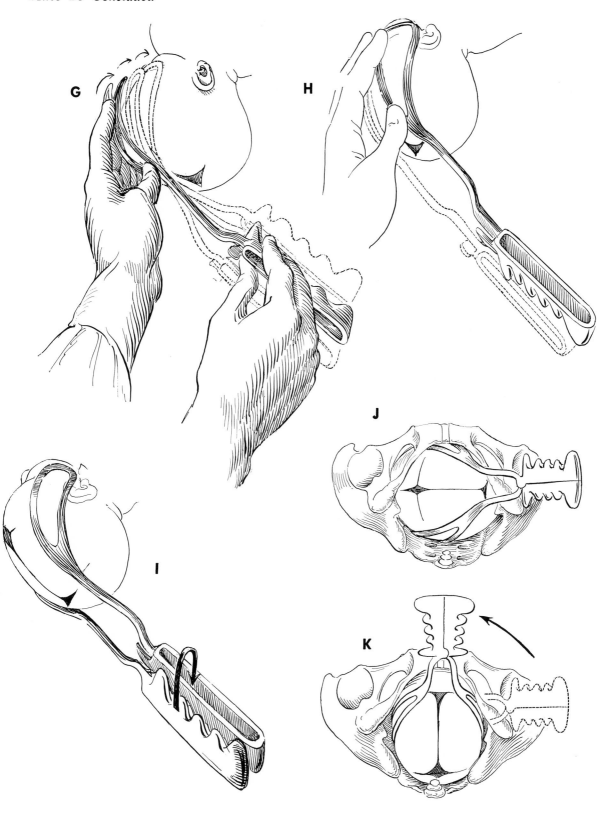

G

H

J

I

K

Plate 24

Forceps delivery—occiput right transverse position

A. The desired application. The sagittal suture parallels the transverse diameter of the pelvis, with the posterior fontanel directed toward the right lateral pelvic wall and the anterior fontanel directed opposite it. The blades are in ideal application in the anteroposterior diameter of the pelvis, with the superior surface of the instrument facing the right side of the pelvis.

B. All four fingers of the operator's right hand are introduced into the left side of the vagina between the infant's forehead and the lateral pelvic wall. The handle of the forceps is grasped in his left hand, and the tip is inserted through the introitus between his fingers and the infant's head.

C. As the handle is swung downward and toward the mother's left thigh, the blade slides around the head between the palmar surfaces of the operator's fingers and the infant's forehead and comes to rest over the infant's face in pelvic application, with its pelvic curve approximating the curve of the birth canal.

126

Plate 24

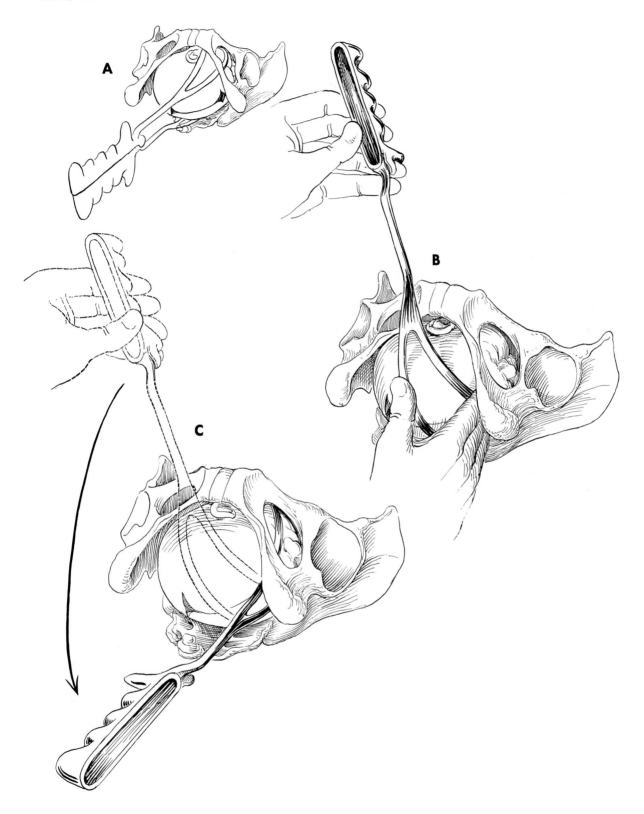

Plate 24 *Continued*

Forceps delivery—occiput right transverse position

D. While an assistant holds the left half of the forceps in place, the operator inserts the tip of the right blade through the right posterior portion of the introitus between the four fingers of his left hand and the parietal eminence.

E. The handle is swung downward and toward the mother's right thigh, and the blade slides into the vagina between the palmar surfaces of the fingers and the right parietal bone and comes to rest in approximately ideal cephalic application, with its anterior surface directed toward the right side of the pelvis.

Plate 24 *Continued*

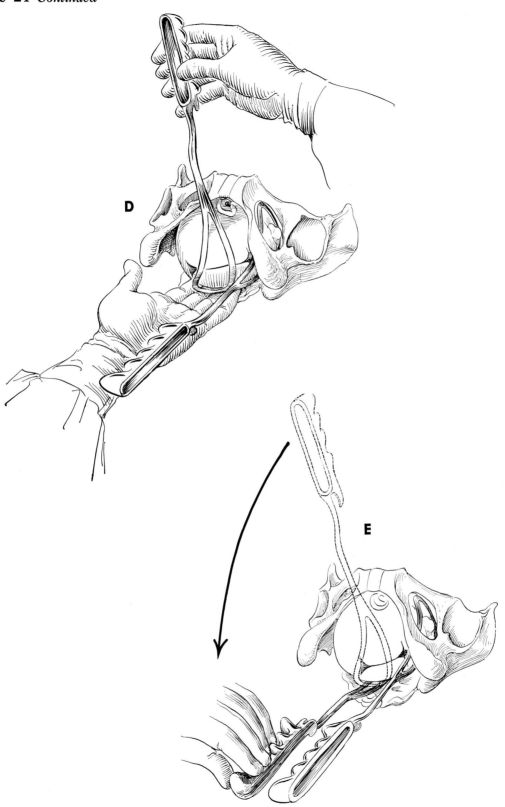

D

E

Plate 24 *Concluded*

Forceps delivery—occiput right transverse position

F. The right (posterior) blade lies in cephalic application in the antero-posterior diameter of the pelvis, but the forceps cannot be articulated because the left blade is still in pelvic application over the infant's face. It must be rotated around the face until it lies beneath the pubic arch in the occipitomental diameter of the left side of the head.

G. The blade is manipulated anteriorly with the fingers and thumb of the operator's right hand while his left hand steadies the handle. The infant's face will not be injured unless it is necessary to rotate the blade forcibly.

H. The ultimate application, with the blades articulated in cephalic application in the anteroposterior diameter of the pelvis.

Plate 24 *Concluded*

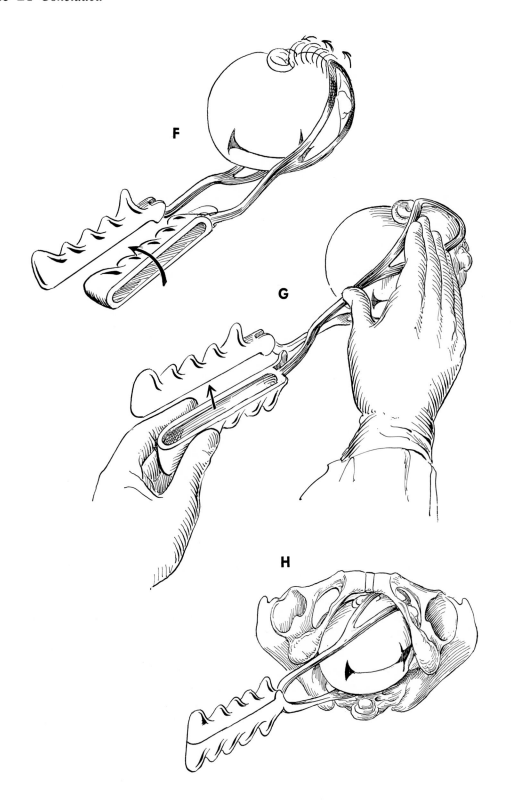

F

G

H

Plate 25

Kielland forceps delivery—occiput right transverse position

Sometimes it is difficult to apply forceps of the Simpson type properly in occiput transverse positions. This is particularly true when the head is relatively high in the midpelvis and in an asynclitic attitude. Under these conditions the operator may obtain a satisfactory application of one blade, but the curve of the birth canal prevents placement of the opposite blade in a position that will permit articulation while it still is applied in a desirable diameter of the head. The design of the Kielland forceps obviates this difficulty.

A. Kielland forceps, anterior surface. The blades are long and have a relatively slight cephalic curve, which makes them more suitable for grasping the elongated, molded head than instruments with shorter blades and a deeper cephalic curve. The two buttons, one on each handle, indicate the anterior surface of the instrument and, with the usual application, point toward the occipital area of the head.

B. The single flange of the locking device is built into the left shank, thereby permitting a mobile articulation. This is in contrast to the English lock, which allows the blades to be locked at only one point.

C. The flange is on the left and the smooth shank is on the right.

D. The sliding lock permits articulation even though the blades are not symmetrically placed with reference to each other. This is particularly valuable when the head is high and is descending asynclitically.

E. The almost complete elimination of the pelvic curve makes the Kielland instrument especially desirable for rotation of the head that is situated high in a transverse position. The head can be rotated to a more advantageous position by simply turning the handles; this cannot be accomplished so easily and safely with instruments with the usual pelvic curve.

F. Forceps in cephalic application in occiput right transverse position.

G. Position of the forceps after 90-degree rotation from right to left.

132

Plate 25

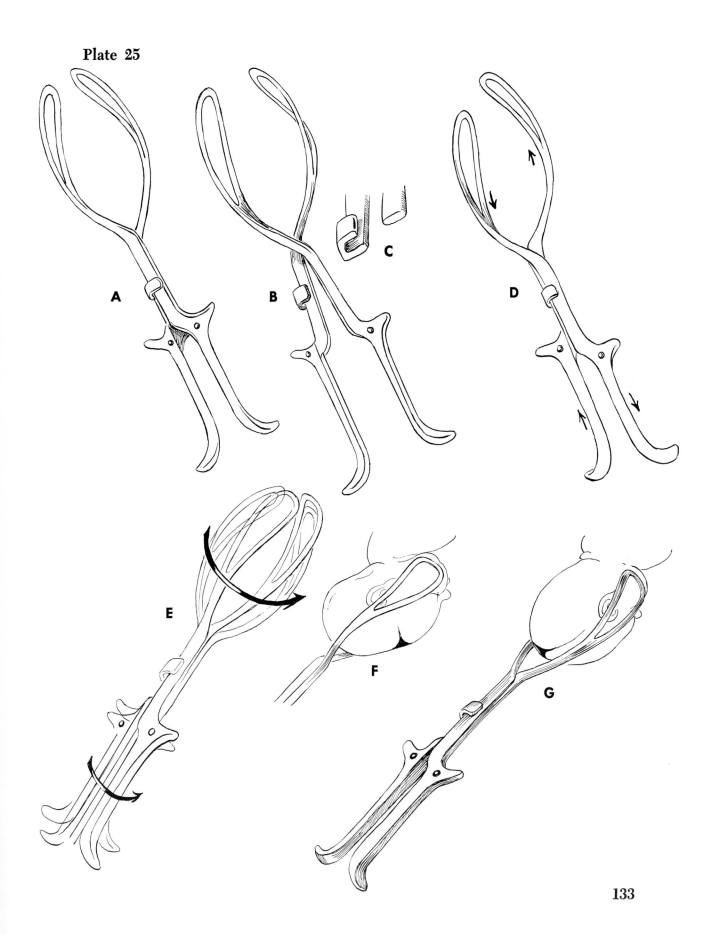

Plate **25** *Continued*

Kielland forceps delivery—occiput right transverse position

H. The desired application in occiput right transverse diameter. The blades are in cephalic application in the occipitomental diameter, with the identification buttons on the handles (anterior surface) directed toward the occiput and the right lateral pelvis. The head is asynclitic, but the sliding lock permits articulation of the forceps even though one blade is at a slightly higher level in the pelvis.

I. Desired application of forceps as viewed from below.

J. The locked forceps are held in front of the introitus in the position they will eventually occupy in the pelvis. The left blade, which will lie beneath the pubic arch in the left occipitomental diameter, is anterior; the right blade, which will lie opposite it in the hollow of the sacrum, is posterior.

Plate 25 *Continued*

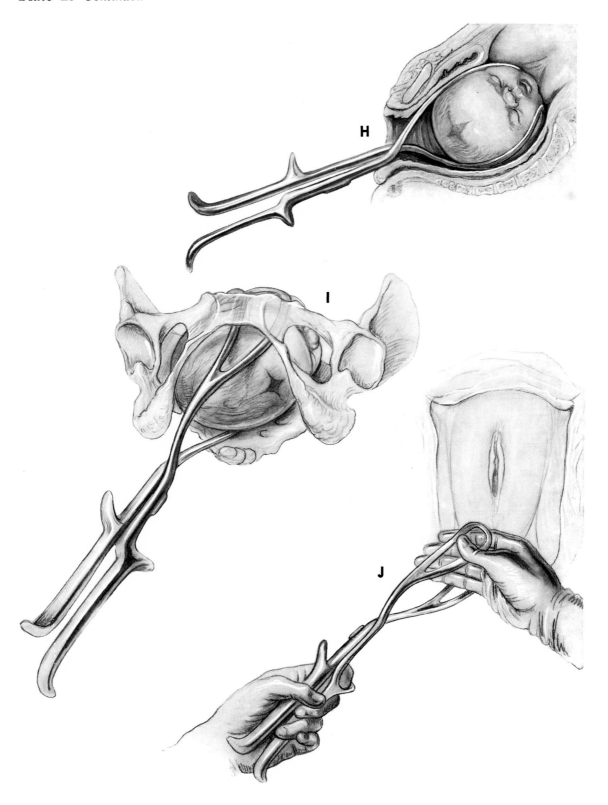

H

I

J

Plate 25 *Continued*

Kielland forceps delivery—occiput
right transverse position

K. The handle of the left half of the instrument is held above the pubis, with the concave surface of the blade directed toward the symphysis and its tip resting on the palmar surfaces of the first two fingers of the operator's left hand just within the introitus. The fingers lie behind the pubis between the left parietal bone and the anterior vaginal wall, and the rim of the dilated cervix.

L. As the handle is swung toward the operator in the sagittal plane, the tip of the blade is slid upward between the fingers and the anterior vaginal wall into the uterine cavity. The cephalic curve points directly anterior toward the symphysis, and the tip of the blade can be felt through the abdominal wall.

The anterior blade can also be applied in the conventional manner by inserting it into the birth canal in pelvic application on the left, with the cephalic curve lying over the baby's face. The blade is then manipulated through an arc of 90 degrees until it lies beneath the pubic arch, with the cephalic curve well applied over the left side of the head. If the dimensions of the bony pelvis are reduced and the head is wedged into the upper pelvis, this maneuver may be more difficult than the usual application.

Plate 25 *Continued*

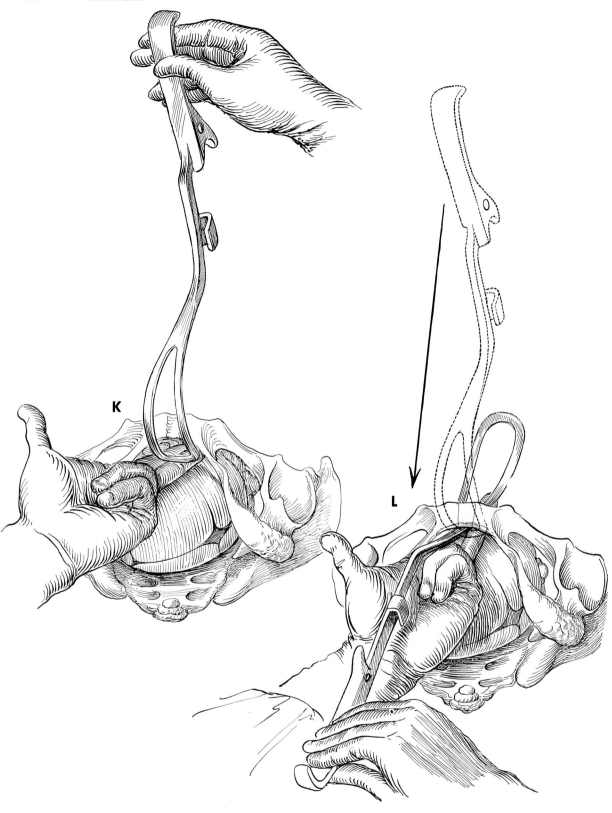

Plate 25 *Continued*

Kielland forceps delivery—occiput right transverse position

M. The blade is now rotated 180 degrees by simply turning the handle, thus bringing its cephalic curve into a position that will permit its proper application to the head. This maneuver can usually be accomplished without difficulty, but if rotation of the blade is forced or if the handle is depressed more than necessary, the tip of the blade may injure the uterus as it is turned.

N. The blade is adjusted by manipulation with the fingers and slight downward traction on the handle until it is properly applied over the left parietal bone.

Plate 25 *Continued*

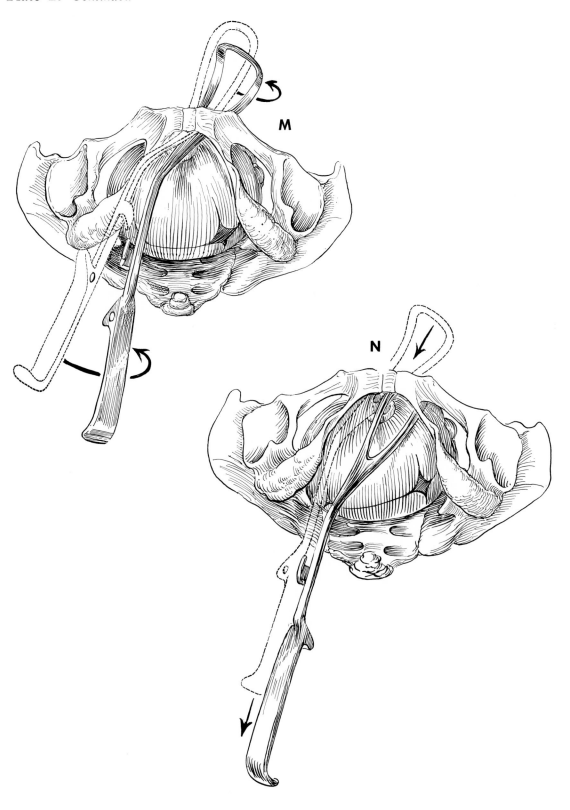

Plate 25 *Continued*

Kielland forceps delivery—occiput right transverse position

O. The handle of the right half of the instrument is held above the pubis, with the tip of the blade resting on the palmar surfaces of those fingers of the operator's opposite hand which have been introduced into the vagina and inside the cervix between the sacrum and the right side of the infant's head. An assistant holds the left blade in place.

P. As the handle is swung downward in the midline, the tip of the forceps glides upward over the fingers into the birth canal until the cephalic curve of the blade lies over the right parietal bone. If flexion is incomplete and the head is high, it may not be possible to apply the blades precisely in the occipitomental diameter, but they can usually be adjusted until they lie close to an ideal application when the blades are locked.

Plate 25 *Continued*

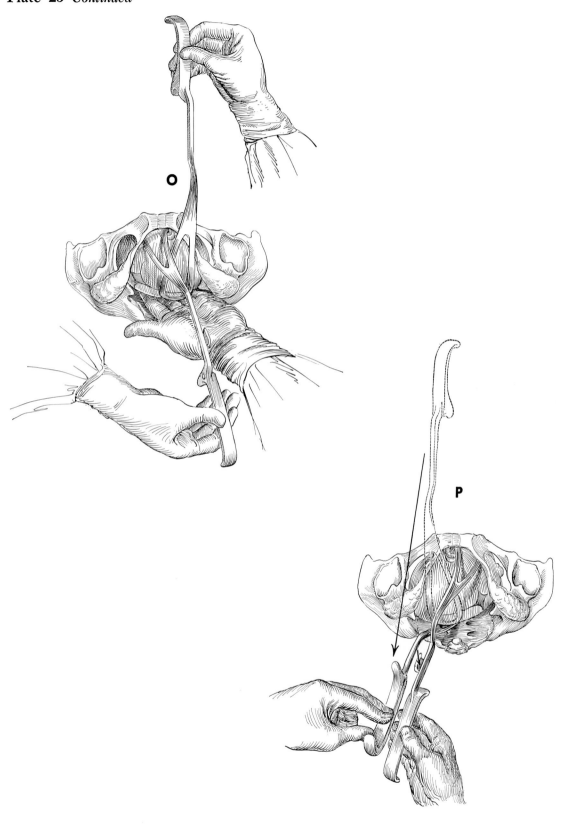

O

P

Plate 25 *Concluded*

Kielland forceps delivery—occiput right transverse position

Q. The forceps handles are grasped with the fingers of both hands, and if the head is to be rotated before traction is applied, it is pushed upward slightly to disengage it.

R. Rotation of the occiput to an anterior position is accomplished by turning the handles of the instrument 90 degrees from right to left. This cannot usually be accomplished unless the head is pushed upward or pulled downward and turned in an area of the pelvis that is more capacious than at the level of the ischial spines. Usually the head will rotate by itself if it can be pulled downward against the converging levator sling and side walls of the pelvis. If the pelvis is flattened in an anteroposterior diameter, as it often is with transverse arrest, it may not be possible to turn the head until it has been brought well down toward the pelvic inlet.

S. The head has been rotated to an occiput anterior position and can now be extracted without adjusting or reapplying the forceps. If the presenting part is still well above the pelvic floor, the most effective traction can be applied by using Pajot's maneuver.

Plate 25 *Concluded*

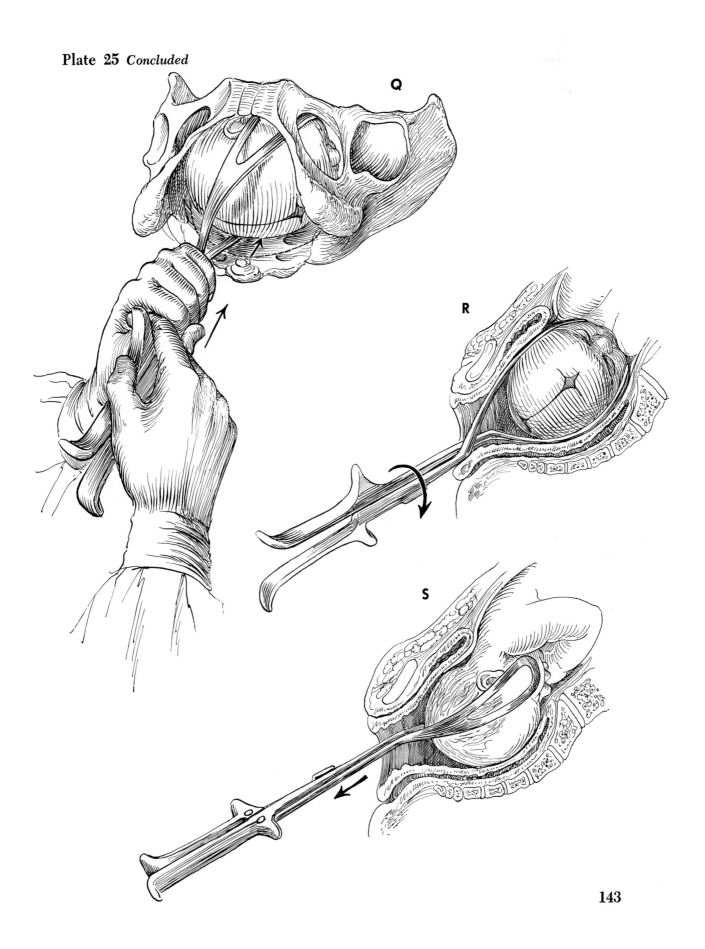

Q

R

S

Forceps delivery—occiput posterior positions

Spontaneous rotation from an oblique occiput posterior position can be anticipated in both multiparas and primigravidas when the pelvic size and shape and the uterine contractions are normal. In others, particularly those with anthropoid pelves or those in whom the infant is in a direct occiput posterior position, the head may fail to rotate but can be expelled without difficulty with its occipital area directed toward the sacrum. However, the operator may be forced to complete the delivery while the head is still in a posterior position if the infant becomes hypoxic as evidenced by an alteration in fetal heart rate or the passage of meconium or if progress in labor ceases despite what appear to be forceful uterine contractions.

Injury to the pelvic soft tissues can be minimized, and pain resulting from the necessary manipulations can be eliminated, by using caudal block, saddle block, or inhalation anesthesia. Pudendal block is almost never adequate.

Plate 26

Forceps delivery—occiput right posterior position

A. The desired application. The sagittal suture parallels the right oblique diameter of the pelvis, with the posterior fontanel directed toward the right posterior quadrant and the anterior fontanel directed toward the left anterior quadrant. The forceps lie in the left oblique diameter of the pelvis, with the left blade over the right side of the head and the right blade over the left side of the head.

B. Holding the handle of the left blade above the mother's right groin with the fingers of his left hand, the operator inserts the tip of the blade through the left posterior portion of the introitus between the four fingers of his right hand and the right parietal bone.

Plate 26

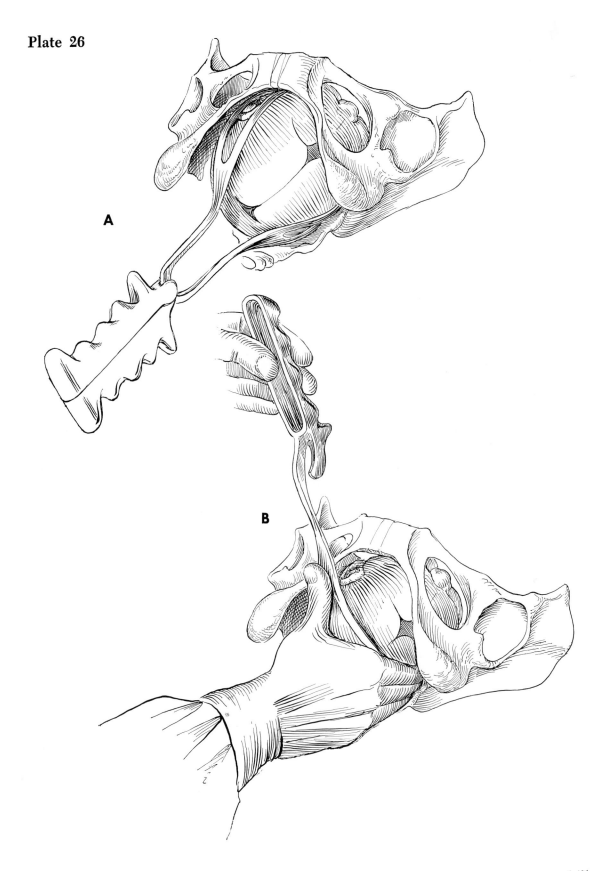

A

B

Plate **26** *Continued*

Forceps delivery—occiput right posterior position

C. As the handle is swung downward and toward the mother's left thigh, the forceps blade will slide upward over the fingers and around the infant's head into the vagina.

D. The blade will lie in the posterior quadrant of the pelvis in the left oblique diameter, with the cephalic curve over the right parietal bone and the cheek of the infant.

Plate 26 *Continued*

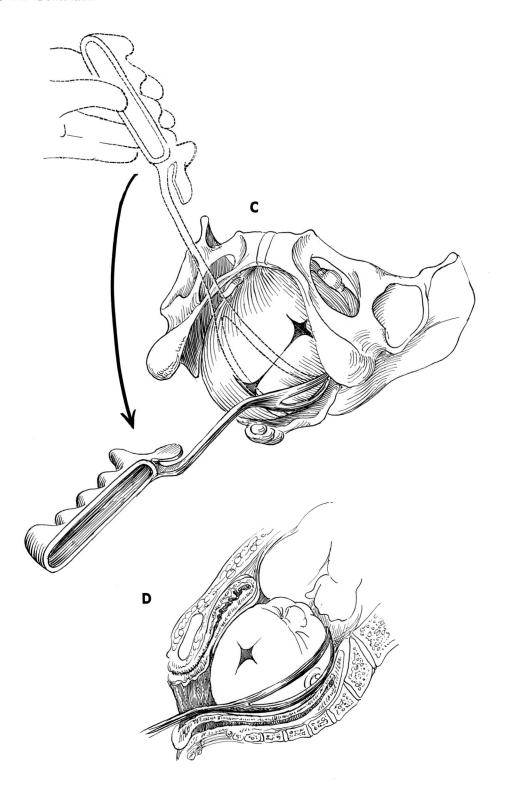

Plate 26 *Continued*

Forceps delivery—occiput right posterior position

E. While an assistant holds the left blade in place, the right blade is introduced by the operator. The handle is suspended above the mother's left groin in the operator's right hand, with the tip inserted through the introitus between the four fingers of his left hand and the posterior portion of the left side of the baby's head.

F. As the handle is swung downward and toward the mother's right thigh, the blade slides over the palmar surfaces of the operator's fingers and around the infant's head until it lies in the right anterior quadrant of the pelvis over the left side of the head.

Plate 26 *Continued*

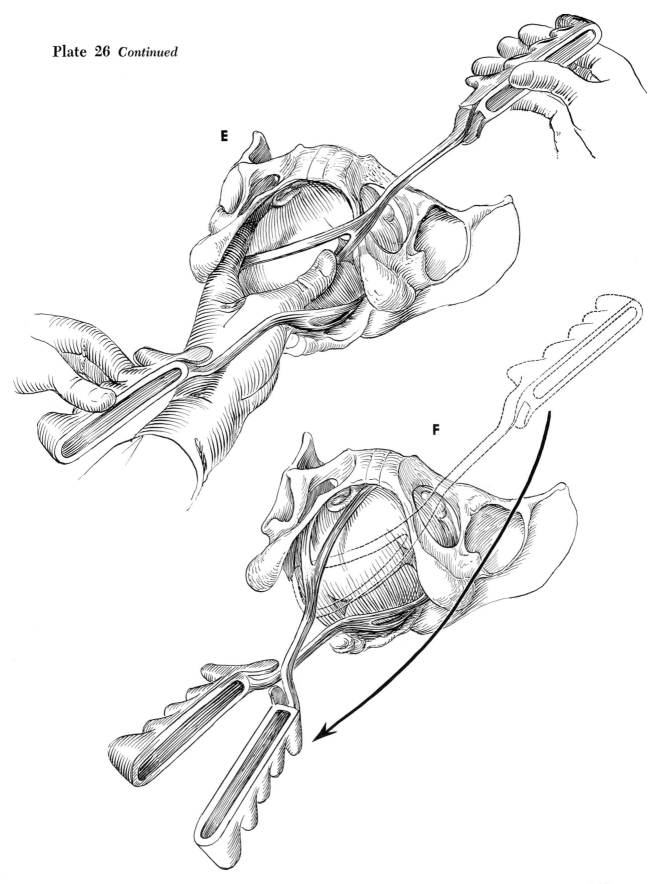

E

F

Plate 26 *Continued*

Forceps delivery—occiput right posterior position

G. The blades are adjusted until they are in proper position over each side of the head and can be locked.

H. As the forceps are articulated, the handles are depressed so that the blades will be applied more posteriorly on the head.

I. The completed application. Flexion of the head can be increased by locking the forceps and raising the handles toward the left anterior quadrant of the pelvis.

Plate 26 *Continued*

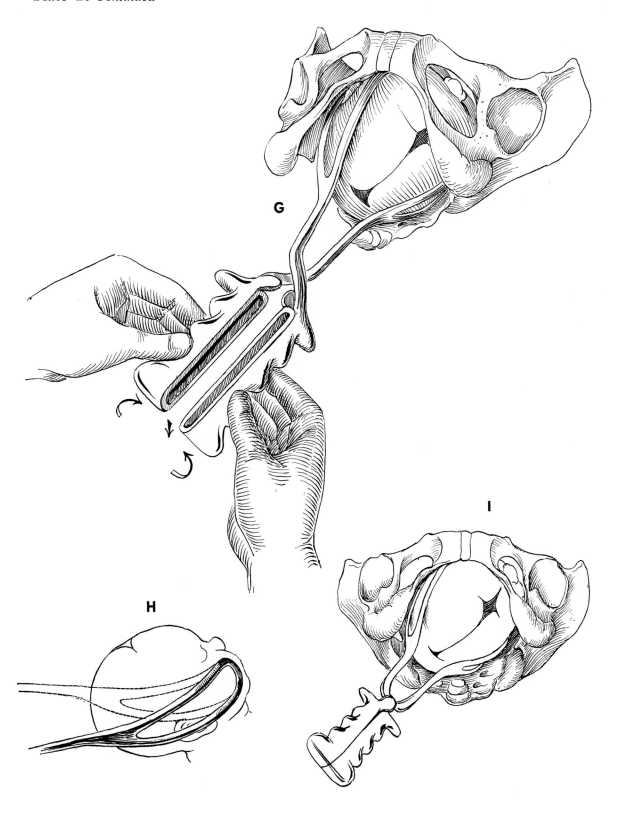

G

H

I

Plate 26 *Continued*

Forceps delivery—occiput right posterior position

J. If the shape of the pelvis and its diameters will permit, the head can often be extracted without difficulty after it has rotated to a direct occiput posterior position. This is particularly true in multiparas. It may not be possible to extract the head with the occiput posterior if the sacrum juts forward and the side walls converge as they do in an android pelvis, but it may be the only practical method of delivering the baby through an anthropoid pelvis if the transverse diameters are too short to permit rotation.

The forceps are grasped with both hands and downward traction is initiated by using Pajot's maneuver. If the head fails to advance with moderate traction, it may be necessary to rotate it before it can come down; however, if it does descend, it will almost always rotate to a direct posterior position as it approaches the pelvic floor, or if not, it can be turned without difficulty.

Plate 26 *Continued*

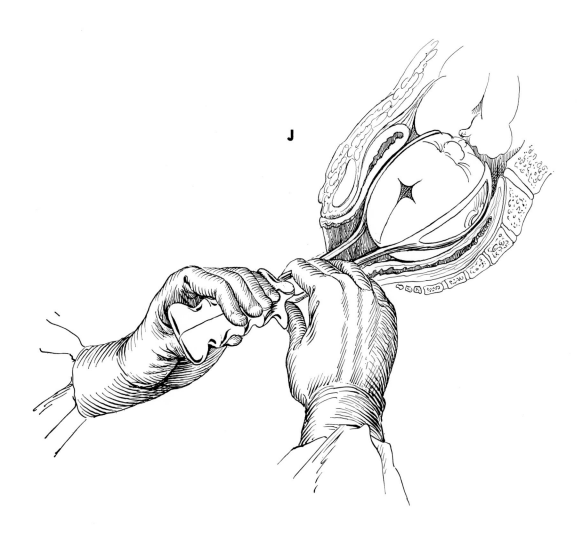

J

Plate 26 *Continued*

Forceps delivery—occiput right posterior position

K. After posterior rotation is complete, the head is pulled downward until the region of the anterior fontanel lies beneath the pubic arch. Because the diameters of the head that emerge through the introitus are longer than those in occiput anterior positions, extensive soft tissue injuries, particularly tears of the sphincter, are likely to occur, and deep episiotomy should be performed unless the structures are considerably relaxed.

L. As downward traction is maintained, the handles of the forceps are elevated. This flexes the head and permits it to follow the anterior curve of the pelvic outlet.

M. Downward and upward traction is continued until the occipital portion of the head clears the perineum and the anterior fontanel can be felt below the pubic arch.

If the fetal head is slightly deflexed and if downward traction is continued until the forehead, rather than the anterior fontanel, lies beneath the pubic arch, the occipitofrontal diameter rather than the suboccipitobregmatic diameter will present in the outlet. Since the former diameter is longer, it may be somewhat more difficult to complete the delivery than when the head is well flexed, and it is more likely that the maternal soft tissues will be injured.

Plate 26 *Continued*

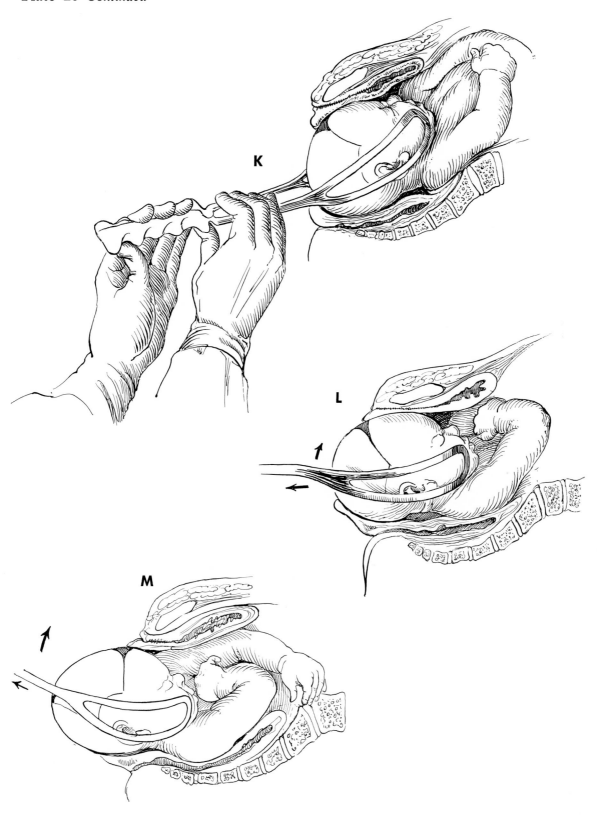

Plate 26 *Concluded*

Forceps delivery—occiput right posterior position

N. The forceps are now removed, and flexion is increased by upward pressure on the back of the head through a sterile towel applied to the perineum. Counterpressure over the area of the bregma will prevent too rapid expulsion.

O. When the occiput has cleared the perineum completely, the head will fall posteriorly as the forehead and face slide out from beneath the pubis anteriorly. From this point the rest of the delivery is exactly like that for the occiput anterior position.

Plate 26 *Concluded*

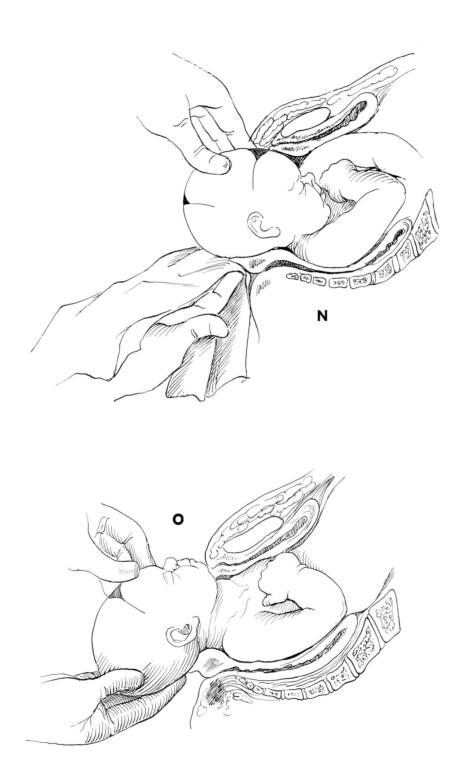

Plate 27

Forceps delivery—occiput left posterior position

A. The desired application. The sagittal suture parallels the left oblique diameter of the pelvis, with the posterior fontanel directed toward the left posterior quadrant of the birth canal and the anterior fontanel directed toward the right anterior quadrant. The forceps are in the right oblique diameter, with the superior surface directed toward the ventral surface of the head.

B. Forceps application in the occiput posterior position. The head may be considerably molded and elongated, and it may be difficult to apply the blades accurately.

C. Ideal application in the occiput posterior position. The maternal soft tissues may be injured if the operator attempts to apply the blades in ideal application because the pelvic curve of the instrument is opposite the curve of the birth canal.

D. After the position has been verified, the handle of the left half of the instrument is suspended above the mother's right groin, with its tip inserted through the introitus between the four fingers of the operator's right hand and the posterior portion of the right side of the infant's head.

Plate 27

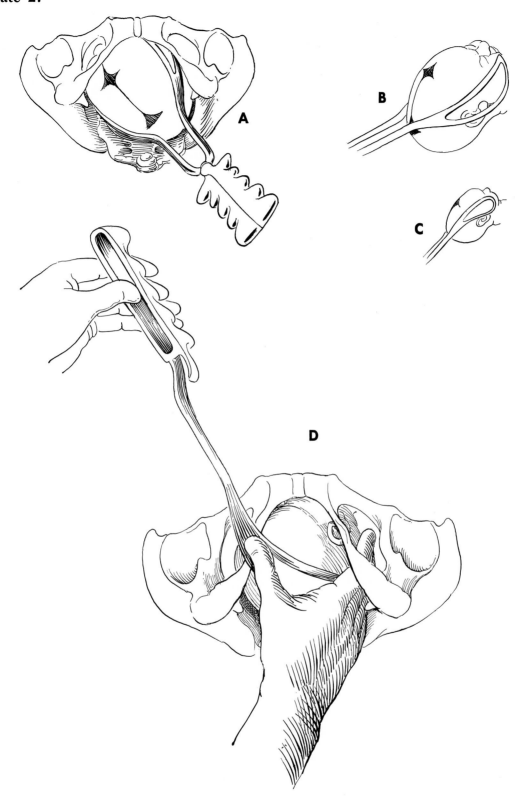

A

B

C

D

Plate 27 *Continued*

Forceps delivery—occiput left posterior position

E. As the handle is swung downward and toward the mother's left thigh, the forceps blade slides over the palmar surfaces of the operator's fingers and around the infant's head until it lies in the left anterior quadrant of the pelvis, almost in the desired position on the head.

F. The handle of the right blade is suspended above the mother's left groin, with its tip inserted through the introitus between the four fingers of the operator's left hand, which have been introduced into the right posterior quadrant of the birth canal (not shown) and the left parietal bone.

Plate 27 *Continued*

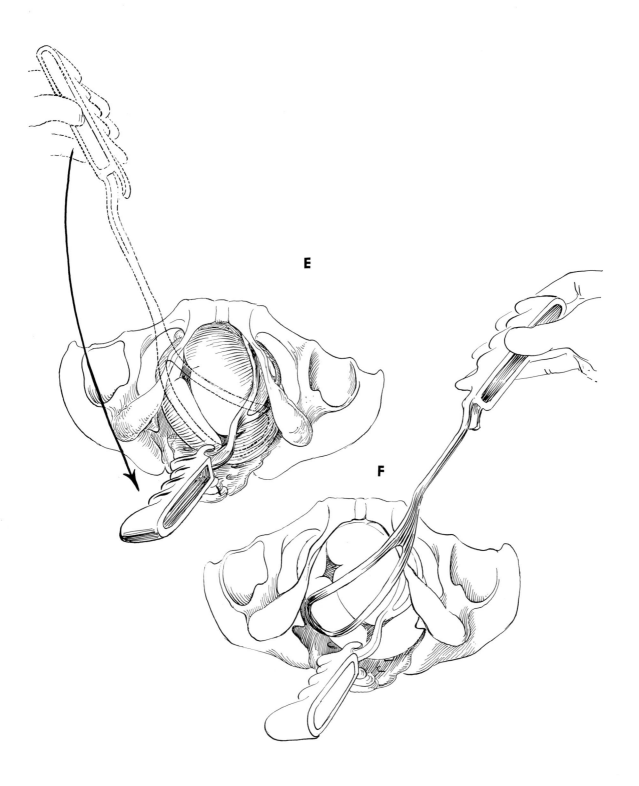

E

F

Plate **27** *Continued*

Forceps delivery—occiput left posterior position

G. As the handle is swung downward and toward the mother's right thigh, the forceps blade slides over the palmar surfaces of the operator's fingers and around the infant's head until it lies in the right posterior quadrant of the pelvis over the left parietal bone.

H. The forceps are articulated as the handles are brought downward and to the left to improve the position of the blades on the fetal head. When they are in proper position and locked, the head can be flexed by elevating the handles. The accuracy of the application is verified by palpating the landmarks on the fetal skull before continuing.

Plate 27 *Continued*

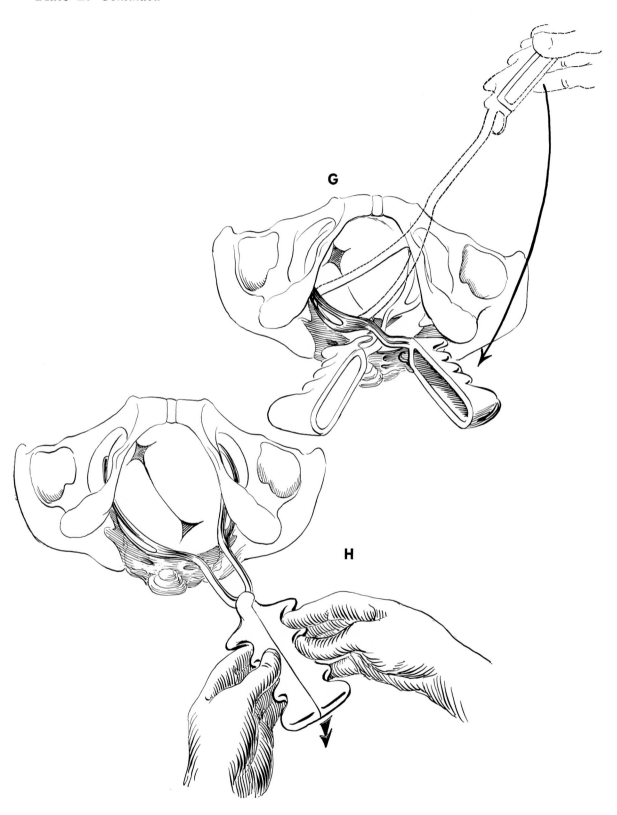

G

H

Plate **27** *Continued*

Forceps delivery—occiput left posterior position

If the presenting part is above the perineal floor, or if the head is elongated, it may not be possible to rotate it without either pushing it upward or pulling it down toward the outlet, because the bispinous diameter of the pelvis is shorter than the anteroposterior diameters of the fetal head. Since many midforceps rotations are made necessary by cessation of descent because of the structure of the mid and lower pelvis, one must usually push the head upward and rotate it above the spines.

I. The head is pushed up slightly to disengage it and is rotated to a transverse position by swinging the forceps handles through an arc of 45 degrees.

J. Anterior rotation is completed as the handles are swung another 45 degrees anteriorly.

K. Correct rotation method. The handles are swung through an arc rather than simply turned over. This permits the tips of the blades to remain in approximately the same area of the birth canal and to serve as a pivot, thereby reducing the possibility of lacerating the soft tissues.

L. Incorrect rotation method. If the handles are turned without swinging them in a circle, the tips rotate through a fairly wide arc and may injure the pelvic wall. This maneuver is permissible when Kielland forceps are used because the absence of the pelvic curve reduces the arc through which the tips of the blades will rotate.

Plate 27 *Continued*

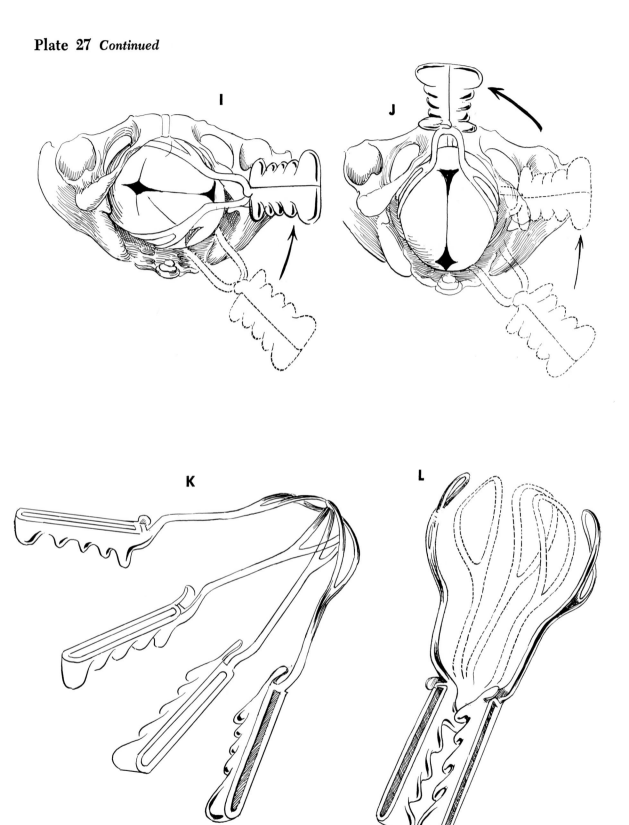

Plate 27 *Concluded*

Forceps delivery—occiput left posterior position

M. Rotation is complete and the head now lies in an occiput anterior position, but the forceps are improperly applied. The pelvic curve of the instrument is directed posteriorly rather than anteriorly, and if an attempt is made to extract the head, the tips of the blades may lacerate the vaginal wall posteriorly. They must therefore be removed and reapplied in a more desirable position.

N. The blades are disarticulated and removed in a manner opposite to that by which they were applied because the pelvic curve now points posteriorly. As the handle of the right blade (now lying over the left lateral pelvic wall) is extracted, it is depressed and swung to the mother's right. This permits the tip to rotate anteriorly as the blade slides around the side of the head, thereby keeping it from lacerating the vagina posteriorly. The opposite blade is removed in a similar manner.

The blades are now reapplied in ideal cephalic and pelvic application, and a forceps extraction is performed.

Plate 27 *Concluded*

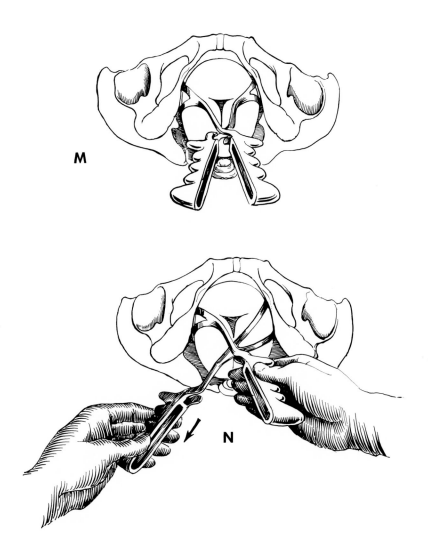

M

N

Plate 28

Manual rotation–occiput posterior positions

It often is easier to rotate the posteriorly situated occiput to an anterior position by manual manipulation than with forceps. If the head can be turned in this manner, the potential injury to the soft tissues that accompanies the original introduction of the blades, the rotation of the head, and the removal and re-application of the instrument can be avoided. If the pelvis is of normal size and shape, the head of a normal infant can almost always be turned without difficulty, and manual rotation should usually be attempted. Even though the posterior portion of the head can be rotated only to an oblique anterior position, the subsequent application of forceps and extraction should be easier.

The rotation can be accomplished with the least difficulty if the voluntary muscles are relaxed and the manipulations are painless; consequently, caudal block, saddle block, or inhalation anesthesia should be administered.

A. Occiput left posterior position. The operator stands facing the perineum of the patient, who is in lithotomy position, and introduces his right hand, well lubricated with green soap, into the vagina. The position is confirmed and the adequacy of the pelvis evaluated. The operator grasps the head, with his four fingers over its posterior surface and the thumb over the parietal bone anteriorly, and pushes upward slightly to disengage it.

B. The head is turned from an occiput left posterior position to an occiput anterior position by pronating the right arm. Because the shoulders are free about the pelvic inlet, they can rotate with the head, and the new position will usually be maintained without difficulty. If the head tends to return to its posterior position, the left blade of the forceps can be applied before the right hand is removed; this will hold the occiput anteriorly until the right blade can be placed in position.

C. Occiput right posterior position. The maneuvers are similar to those described for the occiput left posterior position except that the head is rotated with the operator's left hand from the posterior to the anterior position.

Plate 28

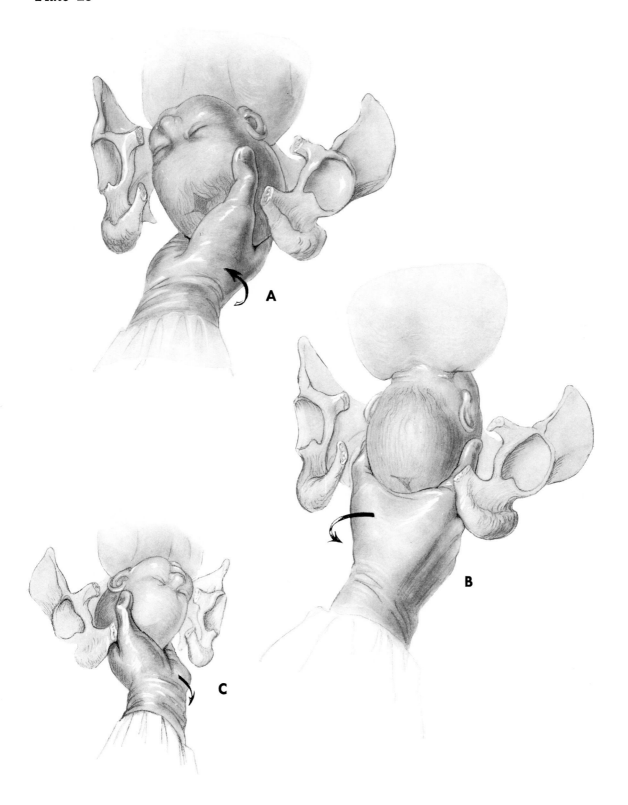

Plate 29

Manual rotation—head and shoulders

When the rotation can be accomplished easily but the head persistently returns to its original position, the operator should suspect that he is rotating only the head while the trunk remains stationary. This is most often caused by the failure of the posterior shoulder to rotate across the promontory from one side of the pelvis to the other, either because it is jammed in position or because the sacrum juts forward more than usual.

A. Occiput left posterior position, with the infant's left shoulder lying in the right posterior quadrant of the pelvic inlet lateral to the sacral promontory.

B. Lateral view of the position shown in A. It is obvious that the shoulder will remain where it is as the head is turned unless a special effort is made to disengage it.

C. To correct the situation and permit rotation of the infant's body as well as his head, the shoulder must be pushed upward and freed. The entire hand is inserted into the vagina (right hand for occiput left posterior positions and left hand for occiput right posterior positions) until the head lies in the palm of the hand and the impacted shoulder can be seized with the fingers.

170

Plate 29

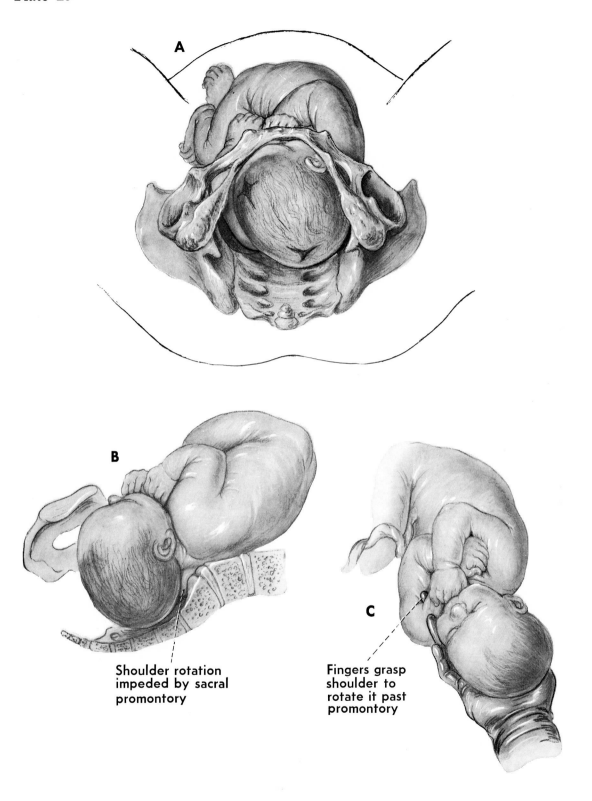

A

B

Shoulder rotation
impeded by sacral
promontory

C

Fingers grasp
shoulder to
rotate it past
promontory

Plate 29 *Concluded*

Manual rotation—head and shoulders

D. The head and shoulders are pushed upward until the shoulder is disengaged from the bony inlet and the head is freely movable.

E. The operator's hand is now pronated, the fingers pulling the left shoulder past the mother's spinal column until it lies on the left side of the pelvis. The head, which of course turns at the same time, now has rotated to an anterior position, where it should remain unless the shoulder slides back. As pressure is applied against the upper pole of the fetus with the hand on the outside, the head is guided back into the pelvis. The hand in the vagina is kept in place until the operator applies the left blade of the forceps, after which it is removed. The right blade is inserted and the infant is extracted.

Plate 29 *Concluded*

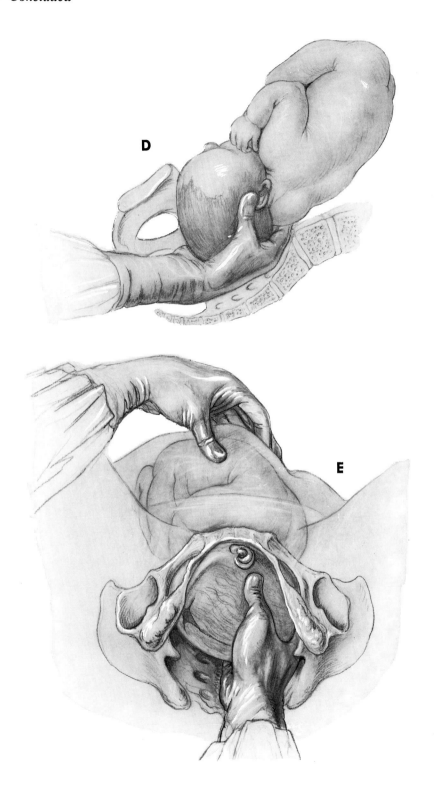

Chapter 8

Face positions

Face positions are encountered about once in every 300 or 400 deliveries and occur more often in multiparas than in primigravidas. Labor usually terminates successfully unless the pelvis is deformed or its capacity is reduced or unless the uterine contractions are abnormal, but delivery may be difficult or even impossible. Infant mortality is increased and may be as high as 15%, the deaths being due primarily to anoxia, injury, and developmental anomalies. Maternal mortality need not be increased.

Plate 30

Face positions

A to G. Although the face positions can sometimes be suspected by abdominal palpation, they are frequently overlooked until the irregularities of the presenting part are felt during vaginal or rectal examination or until the face appears at the introitus. Since the attitude is one of complete extension, the fetal back is concave, and the small parts are thrust forward, being unusually prominent in the mentum anterior positions, **C, D,** and **G.** The cephalic prominence, the occipital portion of the head, lies on the same side as the extended spine and is most easily felt in the mentum posterior and transverse positions, **A, B, E,** and **F.** The characteristic findings may not be obvious if the abdominal wall is unusually thick, if the amount of amniotic fluid is excessive, or if the uterus is irritable.

H. It may not always be possible to differentiate the irregular features of the face from the bony prominences of the breech by rectal palpation, particularly when the membranes are intact, but whenever either is suspected, vaginal examination should be performed. If the cervix is open and the presenting part can be reached with the fingertip, the diagnosis can usually be made. The operator can feel the supraorbital ridges, the nose, the mouth with its sucking action, and the chin unless the landmarks have been obliterated by edema that has developed during prolonged labor.

174

Plate 30

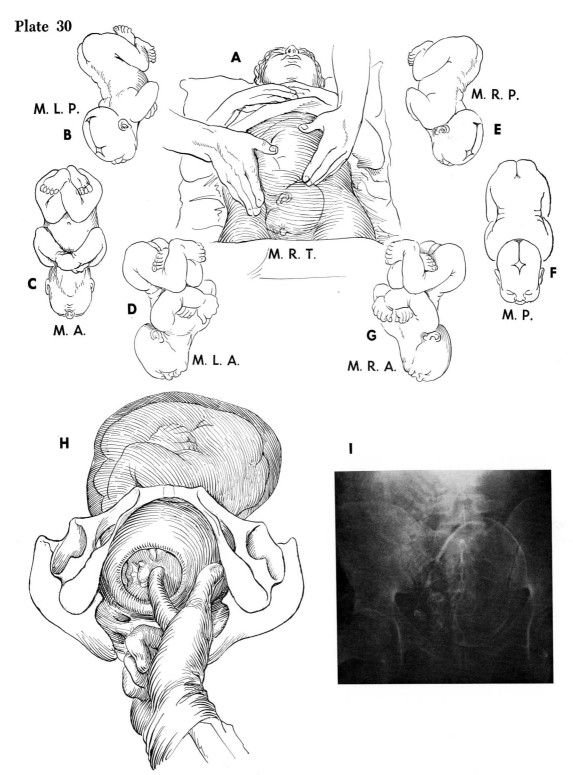

A

M. L. P.

B

C

M. A.

D

M. L. A.

M. R. T.

G

M. R. A.

M. R. P.

E

F

M. P.

H

I

I. The diagnosis can be confirmed by x-ray examination, which is indicated in almost all primigravidas, in multiparas early in labor when the presenting part is high, and if there is any question as to the adequacy of the pelvis. A lateral view is particularly important in determining whether the biparietal diameter of the head can pass the pelvic inlet.

Plate 31

Management of face position

The diagnosis of face position is often not made in multiparas until the face appears at the introitus after a normal labor. In primigravidas, however, the deflexion is usually recognized early. Whenever complete deflexion is suspected on the basis of abdominal or rectal findings, sterile vaginal examination is indicated. If the pelvis is of normal size and shape, if the chin is directed transversely or toward an anterior quadrant, and if the presenting part can be pushed downward to station O or below by abdominal pressure, the operator may anticipate vaginal delivery if the uterus is contracting effectually. However, if the presenting part is wedged into the upper pelvis and cannot be depressed, if the chin is directed posteriorly, or if the uterine contractions are weak and irregular, normal delivery is less likely to occur.

Almost every patient with a face position should be given a test of labor unless the operator can determine by vaginal and x-ray examinations that delivery of the head is impossible. If the cervix dilates and the head gradually descends into the lower pelvis, vaginal delivery can be anticipated. Labor may be slightly longer in primigravidas, but as the presenting part descends to the pelvic floor, the chin will rotate to an anterior position beneath the pubic arch and the head will be born by flexion as the occiput is forced over the perineum. When the face is visible through the distended introitus, the head can be lifted over the perineum with forceps. Episiotomy is almost always necessary to prevent tearing as the long diameters of the head pass through the pelvic outlet.

Occasionally progress will cease before the face has descended to the pelvic floor but after the chin has rotated anteriorly beneath the pubic arch. If cervical dilation is complete and the pelvic outlet is large enough to permit passage of the head, the labor can be completed with forceps. The voluntary muscles should be relaxed with spinal or deep general anesthesia to make delivery easier and less traumatic.

A. The forceps are applied in cephalic application with the blades in the mento-occipital diameter of the head. After the forceps are locked, the handles are depressed to assure complete deflexion of the head, and traction is applied in the axis of the birth canal.

B. When the chin appears beneath the pubis and the perineum begins to stretch, episiotomy is performed if necessary. Traction at this stage is still downward but in a slightly more anterior direction because the face is now passing through the lower pelvis, the curve of which is directed anteriorly. It is at this stage of labor that forceps are often applied electively to complete delivery.

Plate 31

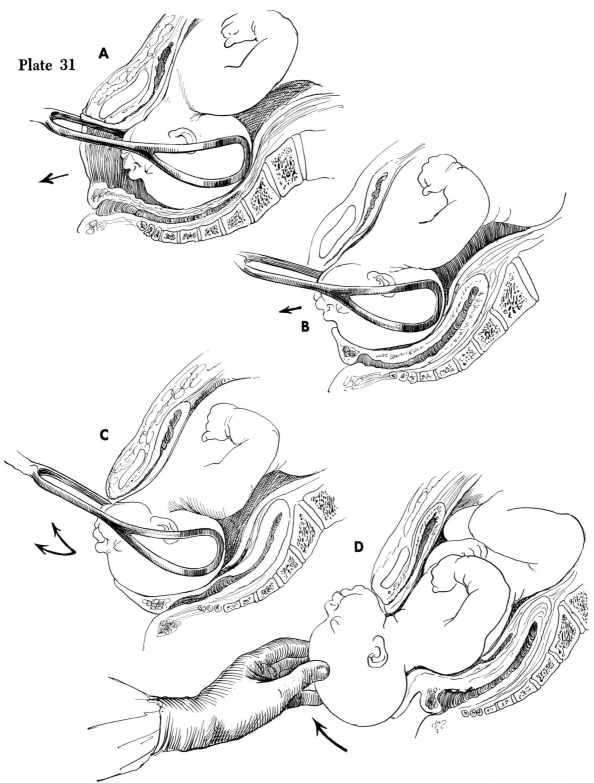

C. With further descent, the entire face and the forehead become visible. The force now is a combination of downward and anterior traction, which results in both descent and flexion of the head as it passes through the introitus.

D. As flexion of the head increases, its occipital portion passes over the perineum and is free. The shoulders descend through the inlet into the pelvic cavity from which they are delivered in the usual manner.

Plate 32

Delivery—mentum transverse position

Labor may come to a standstill before the chin has rotated anteriorly because of ineffective uterine contractions or because the shape of the bony pelvis will not permit further spontaneous rotation or descent. If the cervix is completely dilated, if the chin is at least at the perineal floor, with only slight molding of the skull, and if the pelvis is large enough to permit passage of the baby, vaginal delivery may be possible if the face can be rotated to a more favorable diameter and then extracted with forceps. Unless these criteria can be met, cesarean section is indicated; this is particularly true if the head is high or there is disproportion. The operator must always remember that engagement (passage of the biparietal diameter through the inlet) does not occur until the chin reaches the pelvic floor. Therefore, if the inlet is small, the head may elongate and appear to descend, but the biparietal diameter may be out of the pelvis even though the chin is well below the spines. This can be evaluated most accurately by x-ray examination.

A. After the voluntary muscles have been relaxed with spinal or deep general anesthesia, the head is grasped firmly between the operator's four fingers posteriorly and his thumb anteriorly (left hand for mentum right transverse positions and right hand for mentum left transverse positions). The head is pushed upward slightly to disengage it, and the shoulders and the chin are rotated anteriorly to a position beneath the pubis.

B. Forceps are applied, and the head is extracted as previously described.

Plate 32

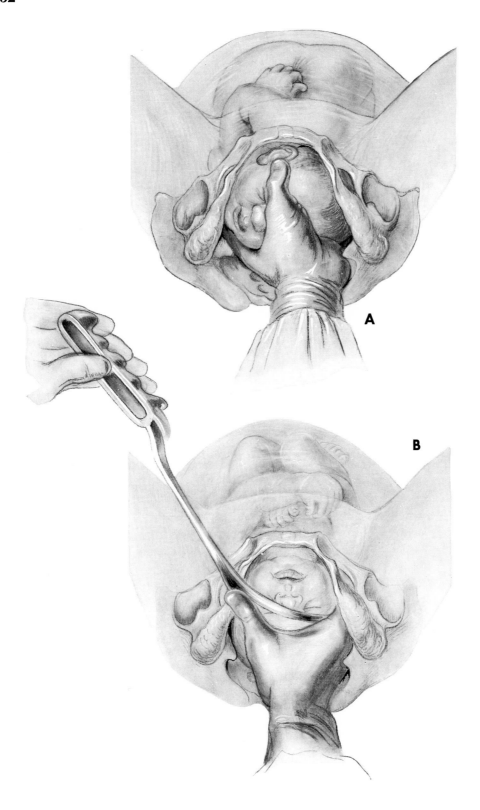

A

B

Plate 33

Delivery—mentum posterior position

If the head becomes wedged into the pelvis with the chin directed posteriorly, vaginal delivery is impossible unless the head can be either rotated 180 degrees or flexed, thereby converting a mentum posterior position to an occiput anterior position. Unless the pelvis is remarkably distorted or the infant is unusually large, rotation of the head often is possible. Conversion to an occiput position can rarely be accomplished because molding is so pronounced when the diagnosis is made that even though the head can be pushed upward above the brim and flexed, it is so misshapen that it cannot be brought back through the inlet. Conversion is most likely to be successful before the head has entered the inlet, but at that time it usually is not possible because the cervix has not yet dilated enough to permit insertion of the operator's hand. Rotation should not be considered unless the presenting part has descended well below the level of the ischial spines, usually to station +2 or +3. If the operator can neither rotate nor flex the impacted extended head, or if the presenting part is still high, cesarean section should usually be performed if the fetal heart rate is normal and no evidence of fetal distress can be detected. If the infant is dead or if its heart rate is slow and irregular, craniotomy and vaginal delivery usually is preferable. Deep anesthesia, either spinal or general, is necessary for all vaginal manipulations. An attempt is first made to rotate the head manually; if this cannot be accomplished, forceps may be tried cautiously.

A. Mentum posterior position from below. The head is completely extended, and the chin is directed toward the sacrum. If the presenting part is still high in the pelvis when the operator decides to terminate labor, cesarean section almost always is preferable to vaginal delivery, but extraction may be possible if the face has descended to the pelvic floor.

B. Kielland forceps are applied in pelvic application over the sides of the head, but upside down rather than in the usual manner.

Plate 33

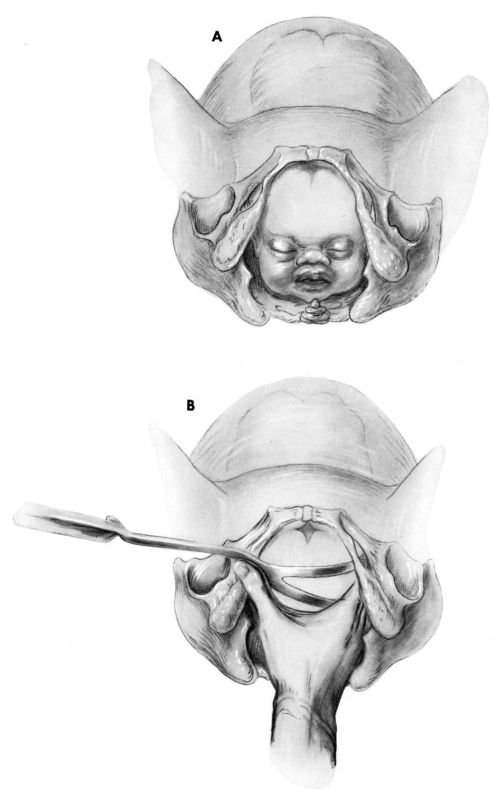

Plate 33 *Concluded*

Delivery—mentum posterior position

C. Kielland forceps are applied upside down, with the buttons on the handles directed toward the floor. Kielland forceps rather than a conventional type are used because they have no pelvic curve and can be applied easily in a position that will permit both rotation and extraction of the head without re-application. The head is pushed upward with the forceps to disengage it, and the chin is then rotated 180 degrees to a position beneath the symphysis. The body usually follows the movement of the head. It is obvious that even though the presenting part has descended deeply into the pelvis, the biparietal diameter of the head is still above the inlet.

D. The forceps are now in the normal position, with the buttons directed upward, and the head can be extracted without removing and reapplying the forceps.

If the head is wedged in the pelvic inlet and does not descend despite strong uterine contractions, cesarean section should usually be considered. A prolonged test of labor is not necessary. The operator can usually determine the eventual outcome after four to six hours of good active labor. Cesarean section is most often necessary for primigravidas, but the operator should not hesitate to perform the operation in multiparas when the head remains high, particularly in the presence of inlet disproportion or mentum posterior positions.

Oxytocin should be used with great caution in patients in whom the infant presents in the face position even though the contractions are of the inertial type. Before the administration of an oxytocic is started, the operator must make certain by vaginal and x-ray examinations that the delay is a result of inadequate contractions rather than cephalopelvic disproportion.

Plate 33 *Concluded*

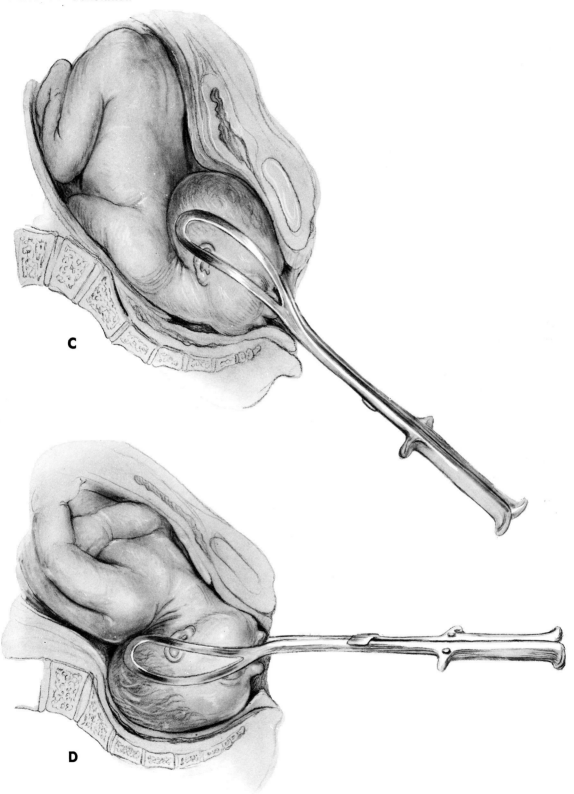

C

D

Chapter 9

Brow positions

When the fetal head is only partially extended, the area of the skull between the anterior fontanel and the bridge of the nose (the brow) becomes the presenting part. Brow or frontal positions are usually transient; the head either flexes to an occiput position or extends to a face position as it descends through the upper pelvis. If the brow position is maintained, as it is in about 0.1% to 0.2% of all deliveries, serious dystocia may develop. The longest diameter of the fetal head, the occipitomental diameter of 13.5 cm., presents, and if the infant is large, the pelvis small, or the contractions weak, vaginal delivery usually is impossible.

Plate 34

Brow positions

A to H. Theoretically, brow positions should usually be suspected by abdominal palpation, but practically, they often are not. The back of the infant is straight rather than flexed as in occiput positions or concave as in face positions, and a prominence is present both anteriorly and posteriorly, **A** and **E.** Small parts are easily felt in the frontoanterior positions, **B, C,** and **G,** and the occipital portion of the head and the straight back are obvious in the frontoposterior positions, **D, F,** and **H.** Obesity, hydramnios, or an irritable contracting uterus may obscure the characteristic findings.

I. The diagnosis can be made most accurately by vaginal palpation. The anterior fontanel can be felt in the middle of the cervical opening, with the sagittal, frontal, and coronal sutures radiating from it. If the head has descended into the pelvis and the cervix is fairly well dilated, the supraorbital ridges and the nose can also be identified.

J. Final confirmation is made by x-ray examination.

184

Plate 34

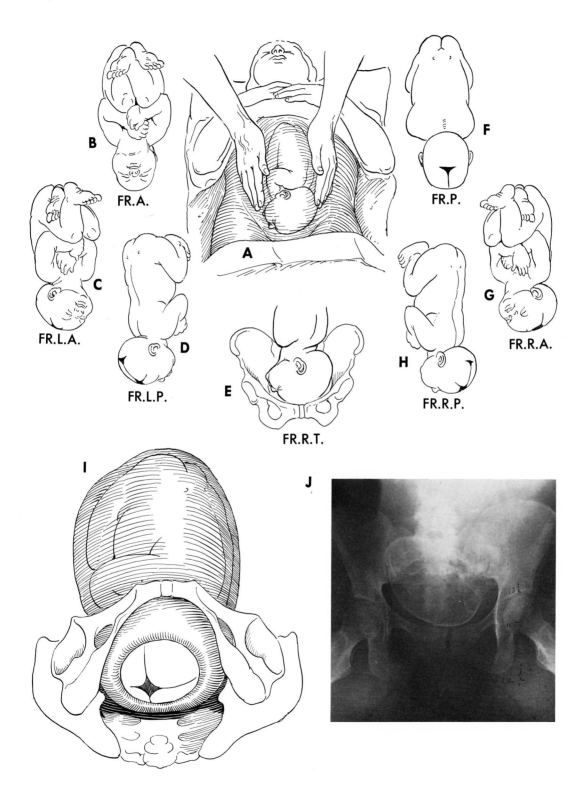

B

FR.A.

C

FR.L.A.

D

FR.L.P.

E

FR.R.T.

A

F

FR.P.

G

FR.R.A.

H

FR.R.P.

I

J

If the pelvis is large or the infant is small, vaginal delivery with the brow presenting may be possible, but spontaneous termination often fails to occur. When a brow position is suspected, sterile vaginal examination should be performed to confirm the diagnosis and to evaluate pelvic size. X-ray pelvimetry should almost always be obtained.

Unless vaginal and x-ray examinations reveal unequivocal disproportion, the patient should usually be given a test of labor. Vaginal delivery can be anticipated if the head descends as the cervix dilates. The head sometimes flexes as it descends through the upper pelvis and eventually delivers in an occiput position. If this fails to occur and descent ceases, the operator may cautiously attempt to flex the head manually if his hand can be inserted through the cervical opening. After the patient has been deeply anesthetized, the infant's head is grasped, with the operator's fingers spread out over the occiput and his thumb over the anterior portion of the skull. It is pushed upward and flexed as pressure is applied through the abdominal and uterine walls and against the infant's chest by the hand on the outside in an attempt to flex the straight spine. The flexed head is then pushed back into the pelvis, and labor is allowed to continue unless the head can easily be extracted with forceps.

If the head cannot be flexed, it is sometimes possible to extend it completely to a face position, which, although far from ideal, is often preferable to the brow position because descent and delivery may be possible.

Attempts to convert the head, either by flexing or by extending it, usually are not successful because by the time the diagnosis is made, the head has already molded to fit the upper pelvis in the deflexed attitude, and it will not reenter in any other position.

Cesarean section is often necessary for the delivery of infants presenting in a brow position and should be considered whenever the head fails to descend after several hours of labor, particularly if one cannot correct the abnormal position. Since vaginal delivery is possible in many women in whom the infant is presenting in a brow position, cesarean section should not be performed until a definite need for the procedure has been established.

Chapter 10

Breech delivery

Breech positions are encountered in the delivery of about 3% of all infants weighing over 2500 grams (5½ pounds) and more frequently in premature infants. Perinatal mortality is higher in breech deliveries than in vertex positions, the main causes of infant deaths being anoxia from a prolapsed cord or from a delay in extraction of the head, injury incurred during delivery, and developmental anomalies, such as hydrocephalus and craniorachischisis, which may predispose to breech positions. It is easy to injure the brachial plexus and to fracture the extremities, particularly if the infant is large. Because of the increased hazard, the family physician should seek consultation whenever he diagnoses a breech position in one of his patients.

Plate 35

Diagnosis of breech positions

A to E. The diagnosis of breech position can almost always be made or at least suspected by abdominal palpation. The smooth, round, firm ballotable head can be felt in the fundus of the uterus, and the smaller, softer, more irregular and pointed breech can be felt over the inlet. There is no cephalic prominence and the buttocks are not ballotable; the fetal heart tones are usually heard best above the level of the umbilicus and are more easily detected when the back is directed anteriorly, **A, D,** and **E,** rather than posteriorly, **B** and **C.**

F. Breech position can be suspected whenever an irregular presenting part is felt during rectal examination and can usually be definitely differentiated from the face or some other portion of the fetus by direct digital palpation through the vagina. If the membranes are ruptured or if only a small amount of forewater is present, the coccyx and ischial tuberosities of the infant can be identified readily.

G. The diagnosis is almost certain when a foot is felt alongside the presenting part, but it must be differentiated from a hand, which sometimes prolapses in front of the head. The anus and genitalia can usually be felt and are easily identified in the male but may be mistaken for facial structures in female infants.

H. X-ray examination confirms the physical findings.

Plate 35

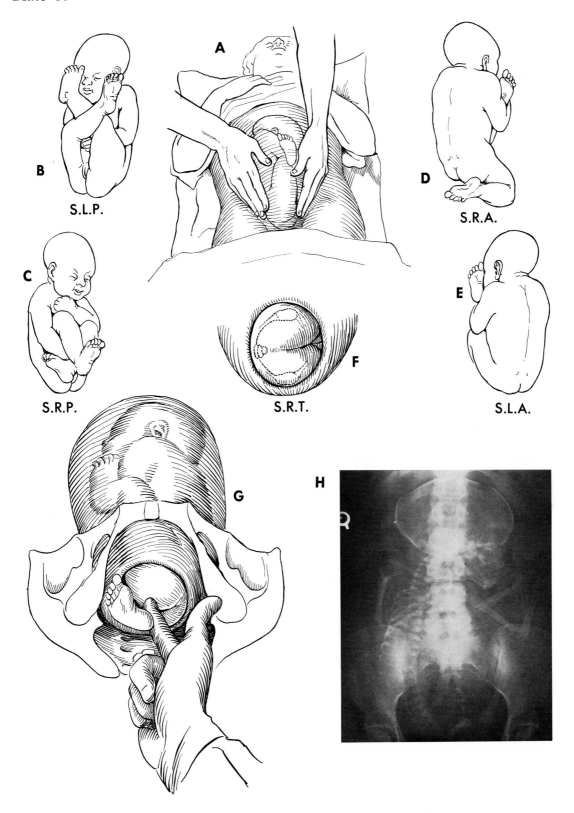

A

B
S.L.P.

C
S.R.P.

D
S.R.A.

E
S.L.A.

F
S.R.T.

G

H

189

Plate 36

Varieties of breech positions

A. Frank breech. The hips are well flexed but the knees are extended, with the feet lying anterior to the infant's face or beneath his chin. It is not usually possible to diagnose a frank breech attitude by abdominal palpation alone, but it can be recognized if only the cone-shaped breech can be felt by vaginal examination. Almost two thirds of the breech positions are of this type.

B. Incomplete breech. In the incomplete breech attitudes, one knee is flexed and one is extended. Since one foot usually lies lower than the other in the complete breech position, these attitudes often cannot be diagnosed accurately by physical examination unless the operator's entire hand can be inserted through the cervix.

C. Complete breech. Both the hips and the knees are flexed, and the feet present with the buttocks. This attitude is easily recognized by digital palpation, particularly after the cervix is half dilated.

D. Knee presentation. One or both knees may precede the breech through the pelvis if the knees are flexed but the hips extended. The knee can be felt below the buttocks when a digital examination is performed.

Occasionally one or both feet present. The hips are usually extended and flexion in the knees is incomplete.

Plate 36

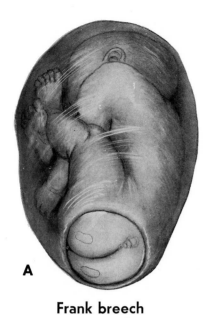

A

Frank breech

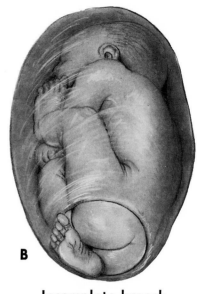

B

Incomplete breech

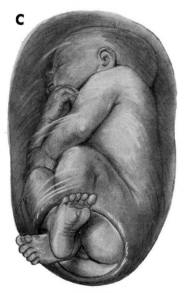

C

Complete breech

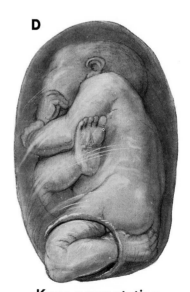

D

Knee presentation

Plate 37

External version

Since the hazard for the infant is increased in breech positions, the end result would be better if the position could be changed. A breech position can sometimes be converted to a vertex by manipulation through the abdominal wall—*external version*. This should usually be attempted first at about the thirty-fourth week of pregnancy, while the infant is small and before the presenting part descends into the inlet; the manipulation can be repeated later if it fails the first time. Version cannot usually be performed after the thirty-sixth week of pregnancy and is possible only rarely during labor.

The main hazards of external version are cord entanglement and separation of the placenta; the latter is usually attached laterally over one of the uterine cornua. Anesthesia obliterates pain sensation and permits too vigorous manipulation. Most of the placental separations during external version occur in anesthetized patients. The operator should count the fetal heart rate frequently while the baby is being turned in an attempt to detect the earliest evidence of a compromised circulation.

A. With the patient in slight Trendelenburg's position, the infant's buttocks are pushed upward out of the pelvis and toward the mother's flank while the head is rotated in an opposite direction. Some authorities recommend that the infant be made to perform a backward somersault, which will help to maintain flexion of the head, but it is more important to turn the baby in the way it goes most easily.

B. The infant is rotated a bit farther. The fetal heart rate should be checked at this point. This is best done with a head stethoscope so that the new position of the infant can be held by maintaining pressure over both the head and the buttocks.

C. The version is half completed. Pressure over the occiput helps maintain flexion of the head. Again the heart rate should be checked.

D. The version is complete.

E. In many instances the vertex position will be maintained, but in others the infant will revert to the breech position. There is no need to apply pressure pads or an abdominal binder in an attempt to hold the head over the inlet, because if the breech position is a more suitable one for the infant, he will re-assume it despite external pressure.

192

Plate 37

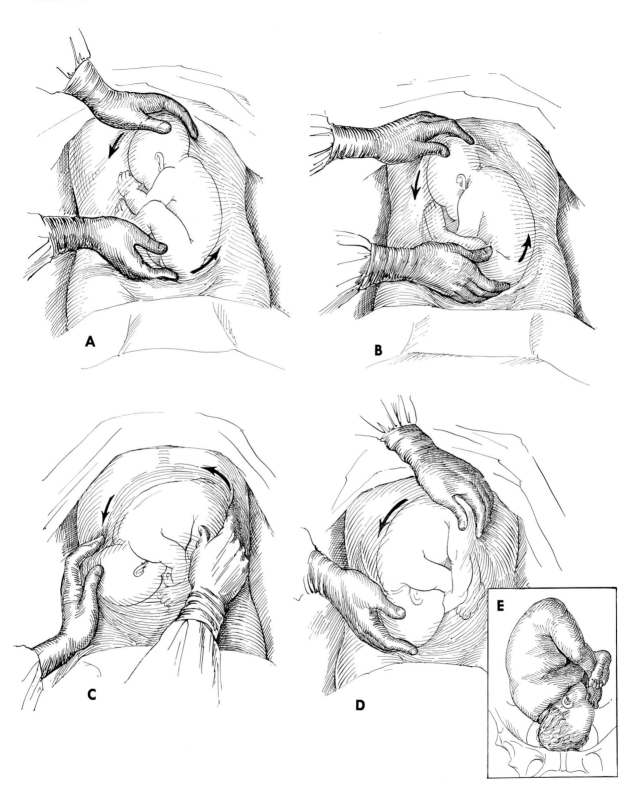

Plate 38

Management of breech labor and delivery

A. When the labor begins, the presenting part usually lies above the level of the ischial spines, with the infant's back directed in an oblique anterior position. The operator should attempt to assure himself by sterile vaginal and x-ray examinations that the capacity of the pelvis is adequate to permit passage of the large unmolded aftercoming head.

B. The presenting part may remain fairly high until the cervix is completely dilated; most of the descent occurs during the second stage of labor. As the buttocks gradually descend, the anterior hip slides up the levator on one side until the bi-ischial diameter lies in the anteroposterior diameter of the maternal pelvis. Intermittent inhalation of a gaseous anesthetic during each contraction can be started at this time, and pudendal block anesthesia can be administered. Saddle block anesthesia has the disadvantage of eliminating uterine and pelvic sensation completely, and the failure to utilize secondary powers may delay further descent of the breech.

C. As labor continues, the anterior hip descends to a position beneath the pubic arch, after which the posterior hip is forced upward over the perineum while the fetal spine bends laterally to accommodate to the curve of the birth canal.

D. Episiotomy is performed when the genital crease becomes visible through the distended introitus.

E and **F.** With further descent of the presenting part, the posterior hip is pushed completely through the introitus. If labor has been progressing steadily, no attempt need be made to extract the infant until both groins are visible.

194

Plate 38

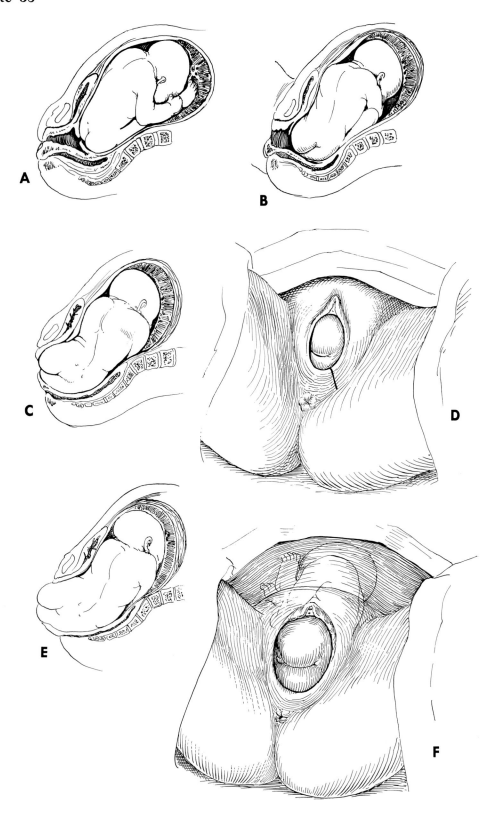

195

Plate 38 *Continued*

Management of breech labor and delivery

G. Downward traction is made with the operator's index fingers in the infant's groins. Pressure should be exerted against the superior surface of the infant's pelvis rather than against the femur; the bone can be fractured, the hip dislocated, or its epiphysis injured by injudicious traction. Inhalation anesthesia is administered continuously from this stage on unless an effective pudendal block has been performed.

H. As the infant descends farther, the traction is directed more anteriorly in the plane of the pelvic inlet.

I. Traction is continued until the knee appears at the introitus.

J and **K.** Flexion and external rotation of the hip are increased by pressure on the femur and the hamstring tendons with the extended fingers. The knee flexes and the foot appears at the introitus.

Plate 38 *Continued*

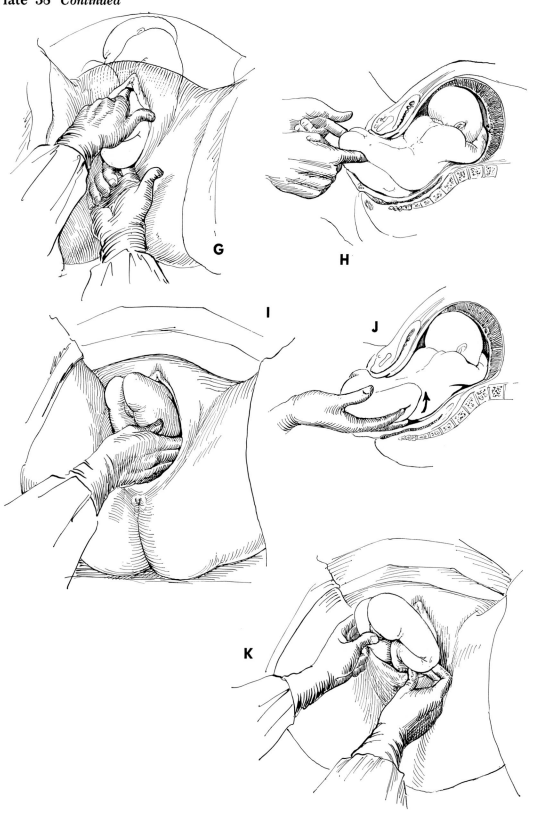

G

H

I

J

K

Plate 38 *Continued*

Management of breech labor and delivery

L. The right foot and leg are now completely outside the vagina.

M and **N.** Pressure on the infant's left thigh increases flexion and external rotation of the hip, and the foot appears and is delivered.

O. Both feet are grasped and pulled downward until the infant's entire pelvis lies outside the vagina.

Plate 38 *Continued*

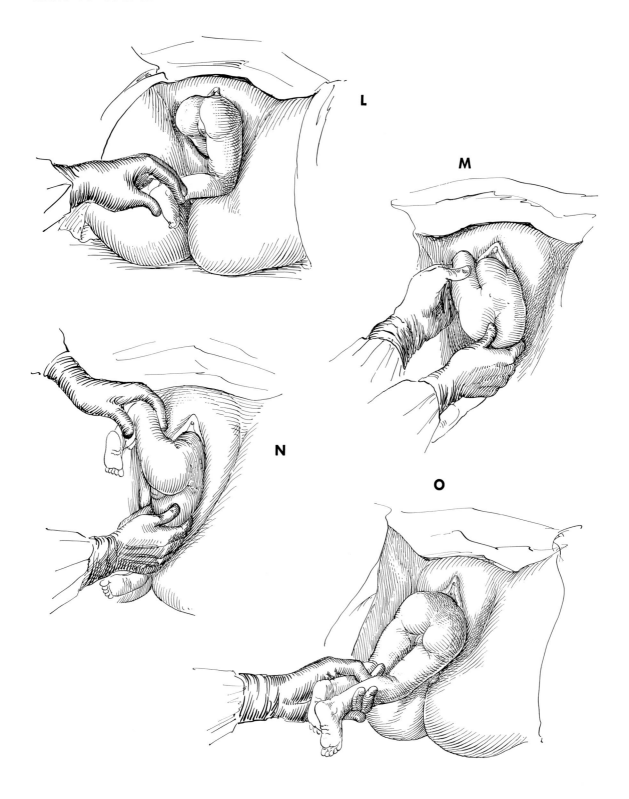

L

M

N

O

Plate 38 *Continued*

Management of breech
labor and delivery

P. Further downward traction is made by grasping the infant's thighs and pelvis, which have been covered by a sterile towel, with both hands. The operator's thumbs lie parallel to the thighs, splinting them, and the tips of his index fingers exert pressure on the brim of the pelvis.

Q. More of the body is delivered from the vagina by continued downward traction. A definite effort should be made to prevent posterior rotation of the back.

R. The anterior scapula appears beneath the pubic arch, while the posterior scapula lies within the vagina in the hollow of the sacrum and is not yet visible. If the arm is flexed across the chest, it sometimes can be freed without difficulty by exerting pressure against the tip of the scapula.

Plate 38 *Continued*

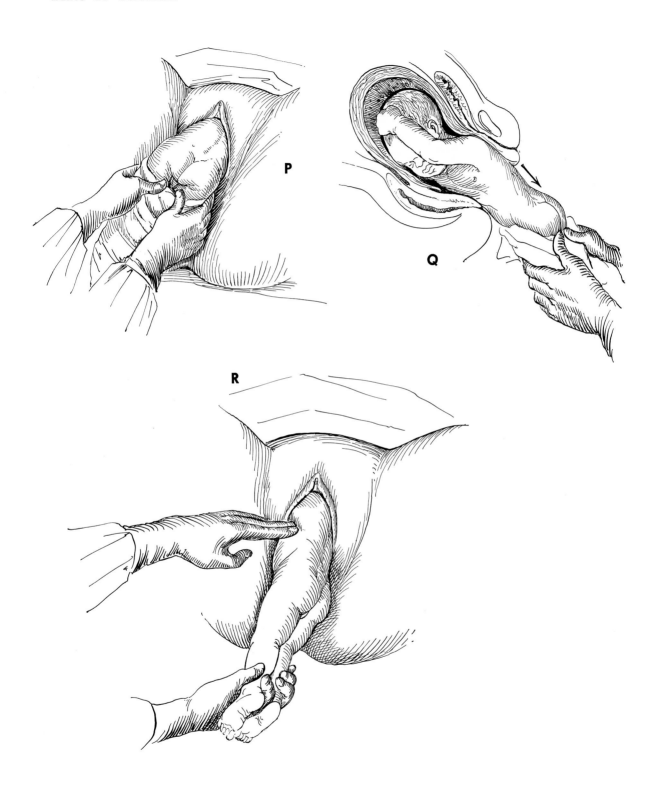

P

Q

R

Plate 38 *Continued*

Management of breech labor and delivery

S. In some instances another maneuver is necessary to deliver the anterior arm. The fingers of the operator's hand (the left hand if the infant's back is directed toward the left side of the maternal pelvis, and the right hand if the baby's back is on the opposite side) are inserted into the anterior pelvis until they lie along the humerus and forearm.

T. The humerus and forearm are swept down across the chest and out of the vagina. The operator must carefully splint the bones and wipe the extremity across the ventral surface of the infant because the humerus can be broken by direct traction on it with a crooked finger.

U. The entire anterior arm has been delivered from the vagina.

Plate 38 *Continued*

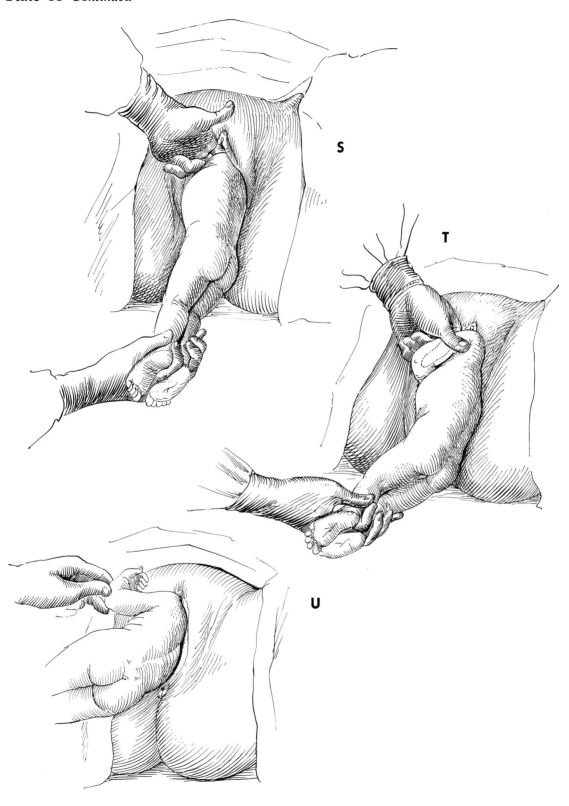

S

T

U

Plate 38 *Concluded*

Management of breech labor and delivery

V. As the infant's body is raised toward the maternal abdomen, the posterior arm may appear at the introitus, but often it is necessary to extract it from its position anterior to the face or chest. The operator's fingers (right hand if the infant's back is directed toward the left side of the pelvis, and left hand if the back is directed toward the opposite side) are inserted into the posterior pelvis until they lie along the humerus and the forearm.

W. The humerus and forearm are swept across the ventral surface of the infant and out of the vagina.

X. An alternative method, which is equally satisfactory, is to rotate the infant's body through an arc of 180 degrees after the anterior arm has been delivered. The arm, which originally was posterior, now lies beneath the pubic arch, from where it can be delivered easily.

Plate 38 *Concluded*

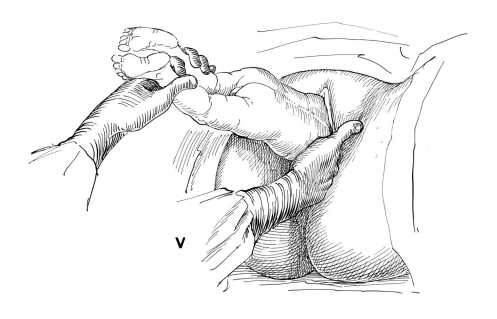

V

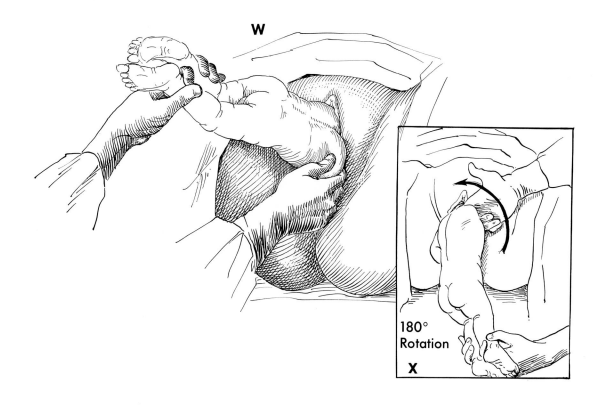

W

180°
Rotation

X

Plate 39

Breech delivery—extraction of head

More babies are lost during extraction of the head than at any other stage of breech delivery. Anoxia develops rapidly because the cord is compressed between the head and the pelvic brim and the infant cannot yet breathe. Unless the mouth is freed within three to five minutes, anoxic brain damage may occur. Because of the danger of anoxia, delivery of the head is often hurried, and with the least delay forceful and frantic attempts, which may be more damaging than helpful, are made to extract it. It is here that an understanding of the mechanism of breech delivery, experience, and ability are of greatest importance, because there is no opportunity to seek consultation, and the operator must know exactly how to proceed.

A. In most instances the head has descended through the inlet and has rotated to an anteroposterior position, **B,** and can be delivered without difficulty, but occasionally it has not yet entered the pelvic cavity. The infant's body is placed astride the operator's forearm, and the tips of the first two fingers of his supinated hand are placed in the mouth or against the maxilla. The head is delivered through the inlet with a combination of traction on the jaw and pressure exerted through the lower uterine segment against the vertex, with the hand on the outside. The head will usually descend most readily with its long axis in the transverse diameter or in one of the oblique diameters of the pelvic inlet. Occasionally another diameter is preferable; for instance, in an anthropoid pelvis, the anteroposterior diameter may be the most favorable. Therefore, when the head cannot be brought into the pelvis, it should be rotated in an attempt to find a more suitable position. If the head is flexed by pulling the chin downward against the chest, somewhat smaller diameters will present, and extraction will be made easier. The operator should never attempt to bring the head through the inlet with forceps, since they rarely can be applied and valuable time is lost in fruitless manipulation.

After the head is brought through the inlet, it usually rotates to an anteroposterior position spontaneously. However, if this does not occur, the face is turned toward the sacrum by traction with the hand in the vagina and pressure applied against the anterior side of the head through the abdominal wall. Since the entire hand and forearm must be inserted into the vagina and through the cervix to perform these manipulations, anesthesia is necessary. The level of the inhalation anesthesia should be deepened when these maneuvers become necessary.

206

Plate 39

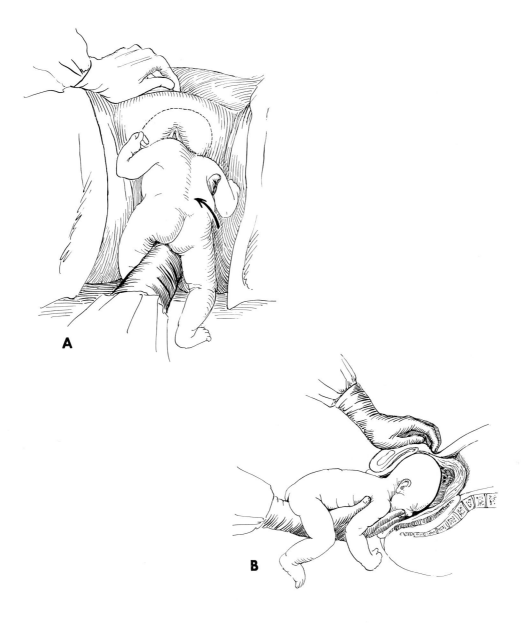

B. After the head has descended through the inlet and has rotated to an anteroposterior position, it is delivered by combined traction and pressure. The force of the traction is at first downward until the mouth appears at the inlet, and then the entire body is raised while flexion of the head is maintained by pulling on the jaw and exerting pressure over the occiput. After the forehead crosses the perineum, the rest of the head can usually be delivered without difficulty.

Plate 39 *Concluded*

Breech delivery—extraction of head

C. If the head cannot be delivered by manual manipulation, it is possible to prevent anoxia by depressing the posterior vaginal wall with a speculum, thereby exposing the infant's nose and mouth. After the secretions have been aspirated from the mouth and nasopharynx, the baby will be able to breathe without difficulty. This will permit careful analysis of the problem and deliberate application of forceps with which delivery can be completed.

In some instances delivery of the head is held up by an incompletely dilated cervix. This is particularly likely to occur during the delivery of premature infants, because the diameters of the head are larger than those of the shoulders and body. When this is recognized by feeling the tight cervix, the posterior lip can often be exposed and incised under direct vision by inserting a posterior speculum. When the cervical opening has been adequately enlarged, the operator can extract the head without difficulty.

Plate 39 *Concluded*

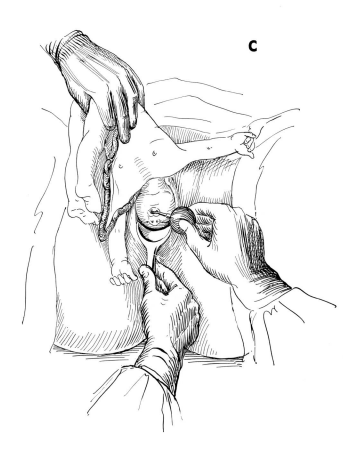

c

Plate 40

Breech delivery—forceps extraction of head

Although the head can usually be delivered over the perineum by manual manipulation alone, forceps extraction is often less traumatizing, and many obstetricians prefer instrumental delivery if the infant is of average size or larger. Forceps extraction of the aftercoming head cannot be performed safely until it has descended well past the inlet into the lower pelvis and has rotated to an anterior position, or almost so. Forceps should never be used in an attempt to pull the head through the inlet or past an incompletely dilated cervix. Either Piper forceps, which were designed specifically to deliver the aftercoming head, or a Simpson type of instrument is satisfactory, but the Piper forceps has certain definite advantages. The pelvic curve is reduced, the shanks are long and curved, and the handles are depressed below the arch of the shanks. All these features make the blades easier to apply to the aftercoming head.

A. While an assistant elevates the baby's body over the pubis to expose the face in the introitus and holds the cord and the upper extremities out of the field, the operator applies the Piper forceps. The arch in the shanks and the absence of the pelvic curve permits the application of the blades beneath the body of the baby directly to the sides of his head. The handles need not be raised over the opposite groin, as is necessary for the application of forceps with a conventional pelvic curve in vertex positions. The first two fingers of the operator's right hand are inserted into the left side of the vagina, and the tip of the forceps blade is passed through the introitus against the palmar surface of the fingers. The handle is held in the left hand below the medial surface of the patient's right thigh.

B. The blade is inserted in pelvic application by sliding its cephalic curve around the side of the infant's head. The right blade is applied above the left blade in a similar manner.

C. After the forceps have been locked, the handles are elevated to flex the head slightly and the infant's body is lowered against the shanks. The head is extracted by pulling downward and raising the handles simultaneously, thereby rolling the face and forehead over the perineum while the suboccipital area remains fixed beneath the pubis.

210

Plate 40

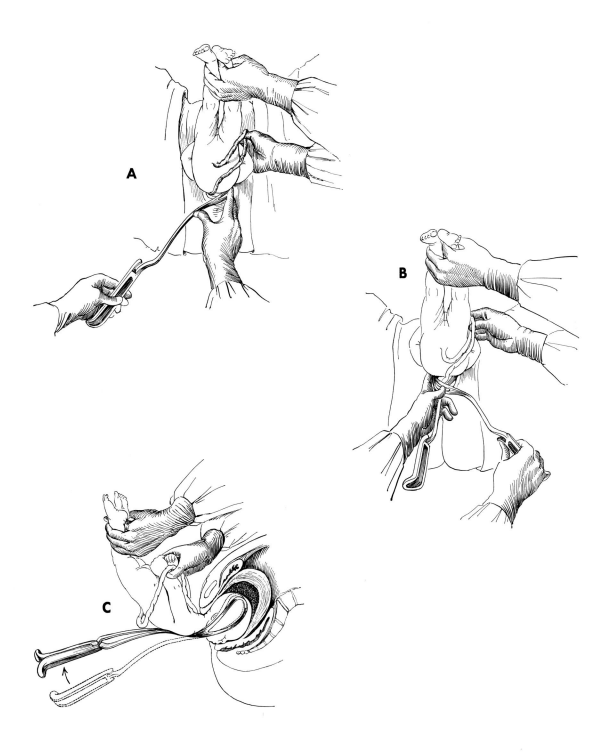

Plate 41

Breech extraction—frank breech position

Complete extraction of the infant in a frank breech position is one of the most difficult and dangerous of all obstetric operations, particularly when performed under unfavorable conditions by an inexperienced operator. Although breech extraction early in the second stage of labor has been recommended as a desirable method for managing most breech deliveries, it should ordinarily be reserved for those patients in whom normal progress ceases. In some instances, the breech cannot descend through the pelvis during the second stage of labor because the extended legs serve as splints that prevent the body from bending to negotiate the curves of the bony pelvis. This is the most important indication for extraction. Delivery may also become necessary if uterine inertia develops during the second stage of labor or if fetal distress, as evidenced by a significant reduction in fetal heart rate, is detected and prompt spontaneous delivery cannot be anticipated. Extraction may occasionally be indicated in patients with heart disease, pulmonary disorders, and hypertension, in whom voluntary bearing-down efforts are contraindicated.

Cesarean section usually is preferable to breech extraction if delivery becomes necessary while the presenting part is still high in the pelvis, if there is any question of fetopelvic disproportion, if an experienced obstetric surgeon is not available to perform the operation, and when the cervix is incompletely dilated.

In order for breech extraction to be performed safely, the cervix must be completely dilated and retracted, the patient must be so deeply anesthetized with an inhalation agent such as ether that intrauterine manipulation does not provoke muscular contraction, and above all the operator must be experienced in breech extraction. The inexperienced physician must always seek consultation before considering this procedure.

A. Frank breech attitude with the sacrum to the left side of the pelvis.

B. The breech is disengaged and the operator's left hand is inserted along the anterior thigh until the index fingertip reaches the popliteal space. If the membranes are still intact, the amniotic sac is perforated at this time.

C. The infant's hip is flexed and externally rotated alongside his body. This maneuver, combined with pressure against the hamstring tendons in the popliteal space, flexes the knee until the lower leg can be grasped with the fingers.

D. The anterior foot and leg are drawn down through the cervix.

212

Plate 41

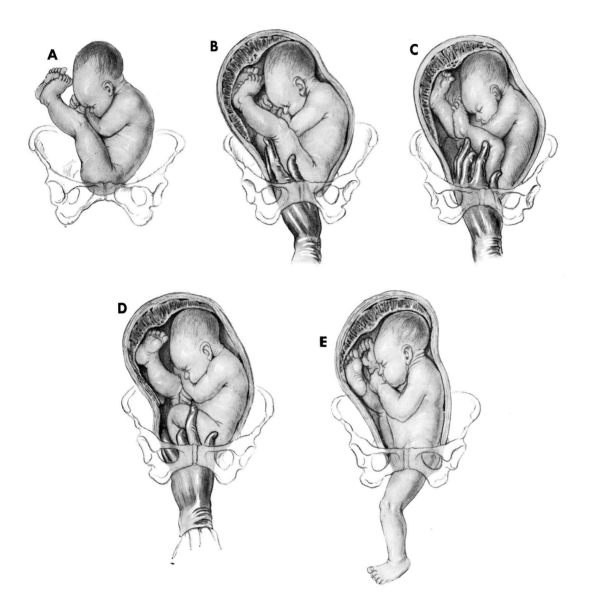

E. Further traction on the leg extends the hip, which now lies behind the pubis. At this time the posterior foot can be delivered in a similar manner, but it is not always necessary. If only one leg can be delivered, the anterior leg should be chosen. If the posterior leg alone is pulled down, the anterior hip, riding over the superior surface of the pubis, can prevent extraction of the rest of the infant.

Plate 41 *Concluded*

Breech extraction–frank breech position

F. The remainder of the delivery is completed as previously described. At this stage the deep anesthesia necessary to perform the intrauterine manipulations is no longer necessary, and the level can gradually be raised. Lightening anesthesia and supplying additional oxygen will be helpful to the infant and will permit the paralyzed uterus to recover its contractile power, thereby reducing blood loss during the third stage of labor. The anesthetic should not be discontinued completely because it will be necessary for the rest of the delivery and is particularly important if the arms are extended and if there is difficulty in extracting the head.

The interior of the uterus should be examined for injury at the completion of the delivery.

G. An alternate method for extracting an infant in a frank breech position is to exert traction on the anterior groin with the fingertip. This may be effective when the presenting part has descended fairly deep into the pelvis, but it is preferable to bring down a leg if the breech lies above the perineal floor. The femur may be fractured or the epiphysis injured by excessive traction on the groin.

Plate 41 *Concluded*

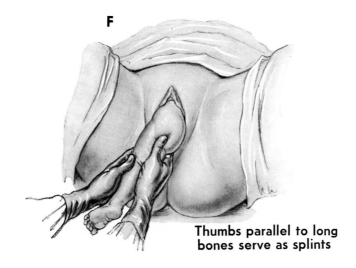

F

Thumbs parallel to long
bones serve as splints

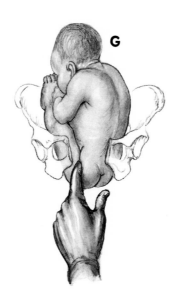

G

Plate 42

Breech extraction—complete breech position

It is far simpler to perform extraction of an infant in a complete breech attitude than one whose legs are extended. The feet usually lie at the same level as the buttocks and, in fact, may have passed through the cervix into the vagina. Little intrauterine manipulation is necessary; consequently, the anesthesia need not be so deep. Either saddle block anesthesia, which relaxes the voluntary muscles and relieves pain completely, or caudal block usually is quite satisfactory.

A. Complete breech attitude, with the back to the left side of the pelvis. The feet lie close together just within the cervical opening.

B. The operator's left hand is inserted through the cervix until the feet can be grasped and pulled downward through the cervix and into the vagina. If it is not possible to bring the feet down together, each foot can be extracted separately, as is done in the frank breech attitude; if only one foot can be delivered, the anterior one is preferable. The remainder of the extraction is performed in the manner previously described.

The cervix should be inspected and the interior of the uterus explored manually at the completion of the delivery because the soft tissues may be injured during the manipulations.

216

Plate 42

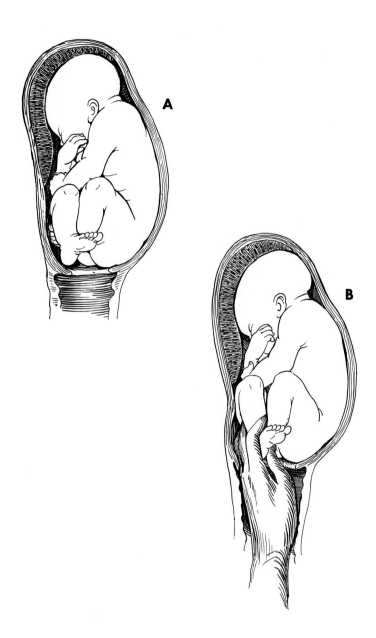

A

B

Plate 43

Breech delivery—extraction of extended arms

During uncomplicated breech delivery, the infant's arms remain folded across the chest, or at least partially flexed, and anterior to his face in a position that permits easy extraction. If the pelvis is small or the infant large, or if the operator attempts to extract the infant too rapidly or to pull the infant through an incompletely dilated cervix, the arms may be swept upward alongside the head. This will delay completion of the delivery, and unless they can be freed promptly, the infant may become anoxic and die.

Extension of the arms can usually be prevented by permitting the buttocks and the trunk to descend through the cervix spontaneously; this will almost always provide enough dilation to permit the shoulders and arms to pass without difficulty. Rapid, forceful traction should be avoided because the arms are so often swept upward during such maneuvers.

Extension of the arms can be suspected whenever progressive descent ceases despite firm downward traction. The abnormality can be recognized without difficulty by inserting the examining fingers through the cervix to feel one or both arms lying between the head and the pelvic brim.

A. With the occiput and the back directed toward the right side of the maternal pelvis, the infant's extended right arm lies between the head and the pubis. The operator's index and second fingers have been inserted until they lie parallel to the humerus. It usually is necessary to push the head and the body upward slightly to provide enough room for the manipulations.

B. Using his two fingers as a splint on the humerus, the operator rotates the infant's forearm anteriorly over the forehead. The arm must be rotated around the head rather than pulled forcibly downward to avoid fracturing the humerus.

218

Plate 43

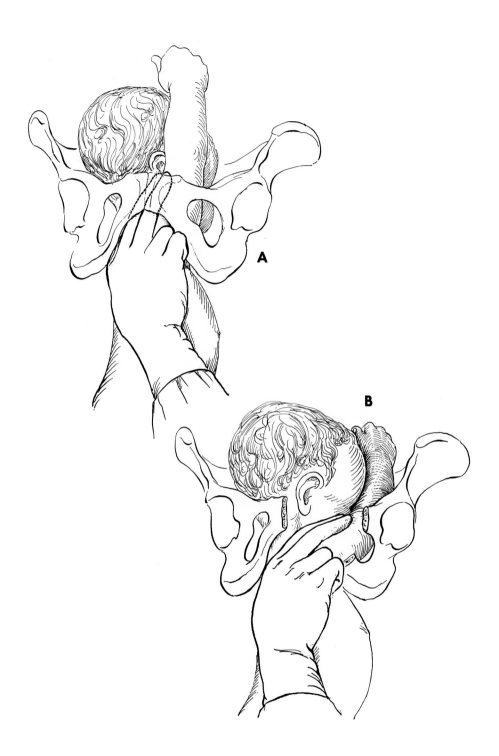

Plate 43 *Concluded*

Breech delivery—extraction of extended arms

C. The forearm is wiped across the chest and finally is delivered in the usual manner. If only one arm was extended, the remainder of the delivery can usually be completed without difficulty, but if the other arm is also extended, it too must be delivered.

The infant's body can be rotated 180 degrees through the anterior pelvis until the back is directed toward the opposite side. When this maneuver is complete, the arm that was extended between the head and the posterior pelvic brim will usually lie anterior to the face, from which it can be extracted without difficulty.

It usually is necessary to insert the entire hand into the vagina to permit the fingers to reach the infant's arms; consequently, good anesthesia is necessary. If an inhalation anesthetic is being administered, it can be deepened as rapidly as possible during the maneuvers. When the infant's arms have been freed, the anesthetic can be lightened.

Plate 43 *Concluded*

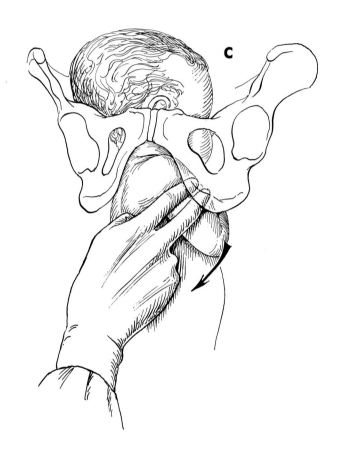

Plate 44

Breech delivery—extraction of arms in nuchal position

Occasionally one or both arms will lie across the infant's neck behind the head in the so-called nuchal position. It is far more difficult to free arms in the nuchal position than those which lie lateral to the head, but it is essential that they be replaced before the delivery can be completed.

A. The back is directed anteriorly, and the operator can feel the left arm crossed over the right arm below the occipital area of the head.

B. The head and shoulders are pushed upward slightly to free them from the pelvic inlet, and the body is rotated at least 90 degrees until the back is directed toward the left side of the pelvis. During the rotation, the left arm will usually be forced into a position of extension behind the pubis and lateral to the head by the pressure from the brim of the pelvis.

C. The arm is wiped downward over the face and chest and through the cervix with the index and second fingers of the operator's left hand.

Plate 44

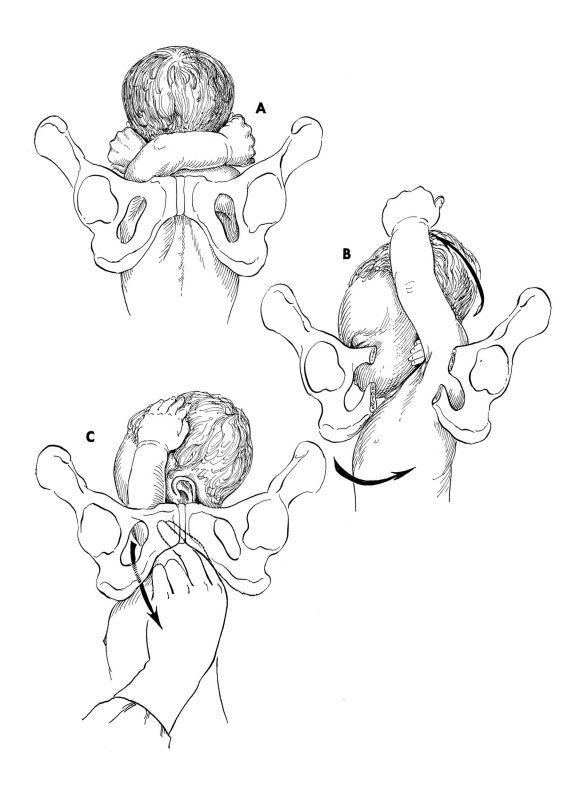

Plate 44 *Concluded*

Breech delivery—extraction of arms in nuchal position

D. The left arm is free, but the right remains in the nuchal position, preventing delivery of the head.

E. As the infant's body is rotated from left to right, the right arm will be forced over the occiput into an extended position. This is the reverse of the initial maneuver.

F. The body and head have been rotated 180 degrees until the back is directed toward the right side of the maternal pelvis. The right arm now lies in front of the face, from which it can be wiped over the chest and delivered with the index and second fingers of the operator's right hand. The head is then extracted in the usual manner.

Plate 44 *Concluded*

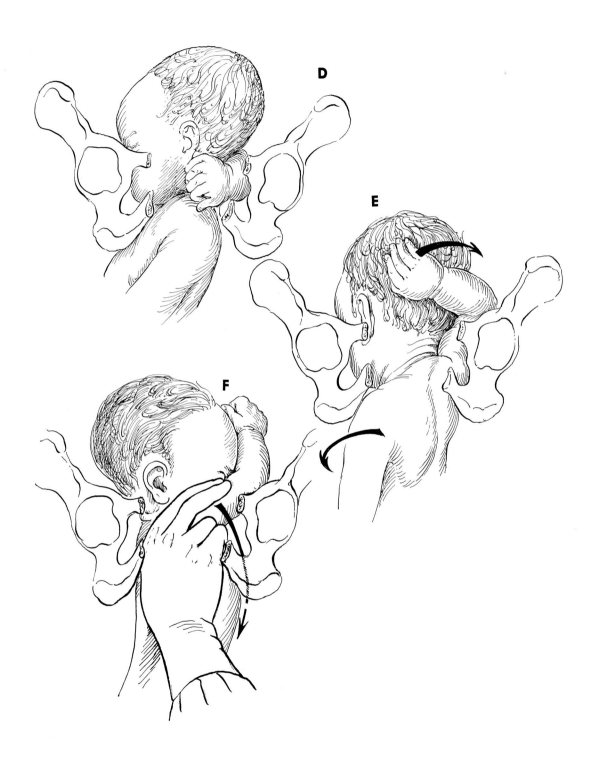

Chapter 11

Transverse lie

In transverse lie, which fortunately does not occur frequently, the long axis of the fetus lies at right angles to the longitudinal axis of the mother's body. Transverse lies are encountered more often in multiparas than in primigravidas. In the majority of patients the length of the uterine cavity is diminished because the placenta is implanted either directly over the fundus of the uterus or in the lower segment; placenta previa is diagnosed in about one third of the patients with transverse lie. Other causes are developmental anomalies of the uterus that broaden the fundal area, and uterine or ovarian neoplasms that prevent the head or the breech from entering the pelvic inlet.

The diagnosis can be suspected whenever the width of the gravid uterus is proportionately greater than its length, and it can be confirmed by abdominal palpation unless the abdominal wall is fat, the uterus is irritable or tender, or an excessive amount of amniotic fluid is present. The head can usually be felt in the iliac fossa or in the flank with the breech on the opposite side; the area over the inlet is empty.

The various attitudes which the fetus can assume in utero are dependent upon the position of the placenta, the shape of the uterus, the size and location of pelvic neoplasms, the amount of amniotic fluid, and the conformation of the infant itself.

MANAGEMENT

Whenever transverse lie is diagnosed during the last few weeks of pregnancy or at the onset of labor, an attempt should be made to manipulate the infant into a more favorable breech or vertex presentation by external version. Although the baby may be quite mobile within the uterus, it will promptly return to its abnormal position if the location of the placenta, the shape of the uterus, or a neoplasm reduces the length of the cavity to any extent. Unless a stable longitudinal lie can be attained, a plan for operative delivery must be developed because successful vaginal termination as a transverse lie is virtually impossible.

Cesarean section. Except under the most favorable conditions, which are not often present with transverse lies, the survival rate for infants near term who are delivered by cesarean section is far better than for those delivered vaginally. In addition, ill-advised or unskillful attempts to perform version and extraction can cause damage to the maternal structures, hemorrhage from rupture of the uterus or cervix or from detachment of a placenta previa, and even death. As a consequence, cesarean section should usually be selected as the preferred method for delivery.

Since placenta previa and structural abnormalities are so often present in women with transverse lie, sterile vaginal and x-ray examinations are necessary when the patient reaches term or as soon as labor begins in an attempt to determine placental location and pelvic configuration. Cesarean section should be performed promptly whenever the infant has a reasonable chance of surviving if external version cannot be performed successfully after labor begins, if the placenta is located in the lower segment, if a neoplasm obstructs the pelvic inlet, if the membranes rupture early in the first stage of labor or before labor begins, if the cord has prolapsed but the fetal heart tones are normal, and in instances of neglected transverse lie when uterine rupture is imminent.

The infant can usually be extracted with the least manipulation and difficulty through a longitudinal rather than a transverse uterine incision, and if the back lies over the pelvic inlet, the incision should be placed in the upper rather than the lower segment. If labor has continued so long that the uterus is tetanically contracted, the lower segment is stretched to the point of rupture, the cavity is infected, the baby is damaged, and the patient is dehydrated and toxic, immediate operation may prove fatal. In most such instances, a delay during which fluids, antibiotic preparations, and morphine or Demerol are administered will make the operative procedure less lethal. Under such circumstances, cesarean hysterectomy usually is necessary, but an extraperitoneal operation may be performed if it is desirable to leave the uterus.

Version and extraction. Vaginal delivery may be possible in an occasional multipara who enters the hospital well advanced in labor with the amniotic sac intact, but the conditions under which version and extraction can be performed with complete success are not often encountered. As a result, cesarean section in the interest of the fetus is usually preferable unless the pregnancy is of less than thirty-two weeks' duration, in which event the chances of the infant's surviving are slight, unless the baby is already dead, or if intrauterine anoxia as evidenced by a consistently irregular heart rate and the passage of meconium can be diagnosed. In such situations, little can be gained by abdominal delivery. Of course, attempted vaginal delivery under any circumstance is contraindicated if the inlet is obstructed or the cervical opening is completely covered by placenta; consequently, whenever this procedure is considered, preliminary sterile vaginal examination is imperative before a final decision can be made.

If the infant is alive and has a good chance of surviving, the patient should remain on the delivery table after the examination, with the responsible obstetrician and a qualified anesthetist constantly in attendance so that version and extraction can be performed as soon as the cervix becomes completely dilated, preferably while the membranes are still intact. The introduction of the largest Voorhees' bag into the vagina or even extraovularly within the lower segment may prevent the membranes from rupturing until complete cervical dilation has been achieved. If the amniotic sac does rupture before the end of the first stage, vaginal examination should be performed at once to make certain that the cord has not been washed down with the gush of fluid. If the cervix is found at this time to be almost fully dilated, the physician may consider performing version, bringing the legs and buttocks through the cervical opening, without attempting to extract. This will prevent the cord from prolapsing and at the same time will permit the contracting uterus to expel the rest of the infant gradually as the cervix dilates, thereby decreasing the possibility of the head's becoming trapped in an incompletely dilated cervix. This is of particular importance in premature delivery when the circumference of the infant's head is larger than that of the other parts of his body. Version without extraction can also be performed to help control bleeding from incomplete placenta previa when the infant is dead or so immature that he is unlikely to survive.

The main hazard for the mother is soft tissue injuries, the most serious of which are rupture of the uterine wall during version and of the incompletely dilated cervix during extraction. The former can usually be avoided if the patient is anesthetized to a depth at which uterine contractions, both spontaneous and those induced by manipulation, are inhibited. This can best be accomplished with ether or chloroform, but cyclopropane is also effective and its action is more rapid. As in breech extraction, the anesthesia can be lightened after the infant has been turned. The uterus will regain some of its tone during the extraction, and bleeding in the third stage of labor will thereby be reduced. The operator should always explore the uterus manually and inspect the cervix and vagina visually after version and extraction, no matter how easily it was accomplished, in search of an unsuspected soft tissue injury.

228

Version and extraction in the management of transverse lie is one of the most difficult and potentially dangerous of all obstetric operations, and unless both the operator and the anesthetist are experienced and skillful, cesarean section is safer for the mother. Because of the possibility of extensive injury and consequent hemorrhage, at least two units of compatible blood should be available when the operation is started.

Plate 45

Various attitudes assumed by the fetus in utero

A. Oblique lie. The long axis of the infant forms an acute angle with the maternal spine rather than approximating a right angle (transverse). Therefore, it is between the transverse and longitudinal lie. Oblique lie is encountered fairly frequently during late pregnancy in multiparas and usually corrects itself spontaneously during early labor. However, if the oblique lie is caused by an obstruction at the inlet, a true transverse lie is likely to develop when the membranes rupture or as labor progresses.

B. Scapula left anterior. The infant's back is directed anteriorly, and the presenting shoulder lies in the left anterior pelvis.

C. The ventral surface of the infant is directed toward the pelvic inlet and the back toward the fundus of the uterus. This position, which is most often encountered in patients with advanced grades of placenta previa, predisposes to cord prolapse because the funis hangs down directly over the empty inlet.

D. Scapula right posterior. The infant's back is directed toward the maternal spine, and the presenting shoulder lies in the right posterior pelvis.

E. The ventral surface of the infant is directed toward the fundal portion of the uterus, and the back lies over the pelvic inlet. The placenta usually is implanted in the fundus, and consequently prolapse of the cord is less likely to occur than when the ventral surface of the infant is directed toward the pelvic inlet and the back toward the fundus of the uterus.

F. Scapula right posterior with prolapsed arm. The arm, of course, cannot prolapse until the cervix is partially dilated and the membranes rupture; consequently, this complication is almost always encountered after labor has been in progress for some time.

G. If the cervix is uneffaced and undilated and the membranes are intact, the operator usually cannot reach the presenting part through the vagina; however, if labor has begun, the structures can often be identified. The shoulder, the scapula, and the rib cage can be felt through the dilated cervix by the experienced examiner, but it is not always easy to differentiate these structures from the irregular contours of the breech. Because placenta previa is so often present, vaginal examination in patients with transverse lies should be performed in the hospital delivery room rather than in the physician's office, where facilities for control of bleeding and replacement of blood are not available.

H. The most accurate appraisal of the position as well as the size of the baby can be made by x-ray examination.

Plate 45

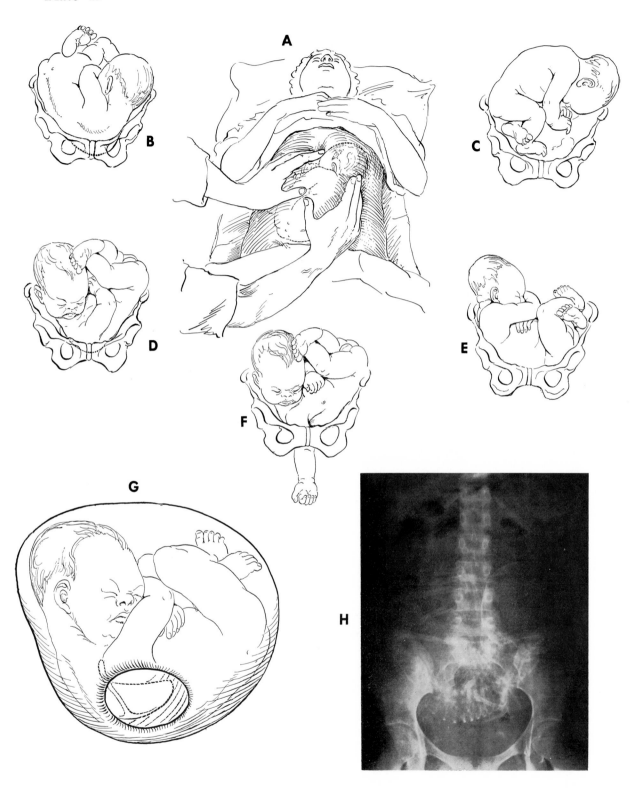

Plate 46

Version in ventral presentation

Version is much less complicated when the ventral surface of the infant is directed toward the pelvic inlet because the feet can be grasped with little intrauterine manipulation. This situation is likely to be present when the baby is immature and there is an excess of fluid, but unfortunately it also is frequently encountered in patients with the more advanced grades of placenta previa when version is contraindicated. Since less manipulation is required when the feet lie just above the cervical opening, the risk to the mother is reduced. Nevertheless the danger can be minimized by adequate anesthesia.

A. The operator's hand and forearm, well lubricated with green soap and encased in an elbow-length glove, are introduced through the vagina and the cervix into the uterus and the exact position and attitude of the infant determined. If the membranes are still intact, the initial palpatory maneuvers are carried out through the sac, which is then perforated with the fingers. The feet are then grasped. It is of great importance that small parts be positively identified before they are pulled through the cervix, because the extraction of both hands or a hand and a foot rather than both feet may complicate the procedure immeasurably.

B. As the feet are pulled downward through the cervix and vagina, the buttocks will follow and the head will automatically assume a position in the fundus of the uterus. It usually is not necessary to apply external pressure in an attempt to push the head upward. The version is now complete, and if extraction is to follow, it is performed exactly as for primary breech positions.

Plate 46

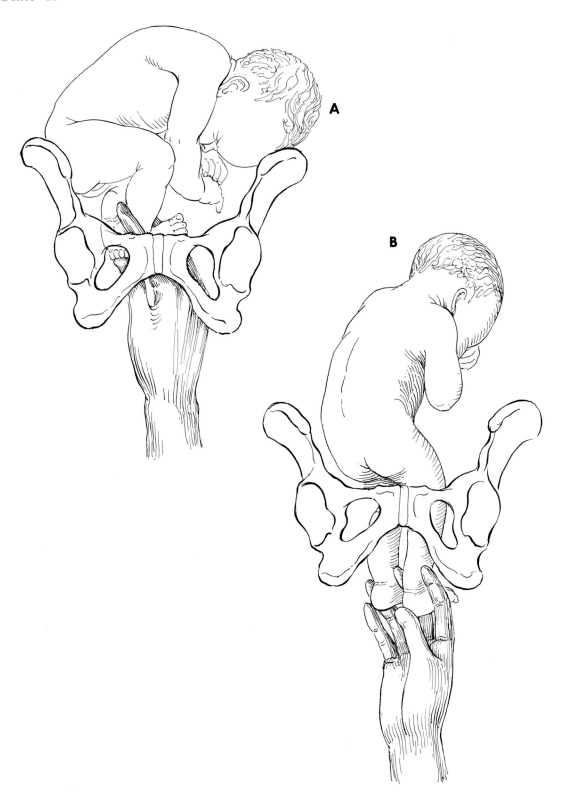

A

B

Plate 47

Version in scapula left anterior position

Version is much more difficult and dangerous when the infant's shoulder is jammed into the pelvis than when the ventral surface of the infant presents. The operator's hand must be introduced deeper into the uterus to reach the feet, and far more manipulation is required to rotate the back upward and to correct the transverse lie simultaneously than simply to pull down the feet. In addition, the arm may be prolapsed and the uterus thin. Here deep anesthesia is of utmost importance. An intravenous infusion of saline solution should be running through a securely placed intravenous catheter before the operation is begun so that blood may be introduced promptly if the uterus is ruptured or excessive bleeding occurs.

A. After the uterus is completely relaxed, the presenting shoulder is pushed upward well out of the pelvis and an exact diagnosis of position and attitude made. Either hand may be used. Some operators prefer to use the left hand for scapula left positions and the right hand for scapula right positions. Since the head usually rises without help as the breech is brought down, the preferred hand is the one that can grasp the feet most readily and carry out the necessary manipulations most effectively.

B. The operator's hand is inserted behind the infant and past the brim of the pelvis, separating the membranes if they are still intact, until the feet can be felt. With his fingers, he then perforates the amniotic sac and grasps the feet—both if possible. If not, it is preferable to grasp the anterior foot, because the infant's back can be most effectively rotated upward by pulling the left leg downward through the posterior pelvis into the vagina. It is obvious that the uterus must be completely relaxed and the shoulder free from the bony pelvis to permit the performance of this maneuver.

C. As traction is exerted on the feet, the back, which was directed toward the anterior wall of the uterus, is rotated through an arc of approximately 90 degrees. The ventral surface of the infant's body now lies above the pelvic inlet, and the feet are directly over the dilated cervix or in the upper vagina. The delivery is completed by the same maneuvers described for ventral presentation of the fetus.

234

Plate 47

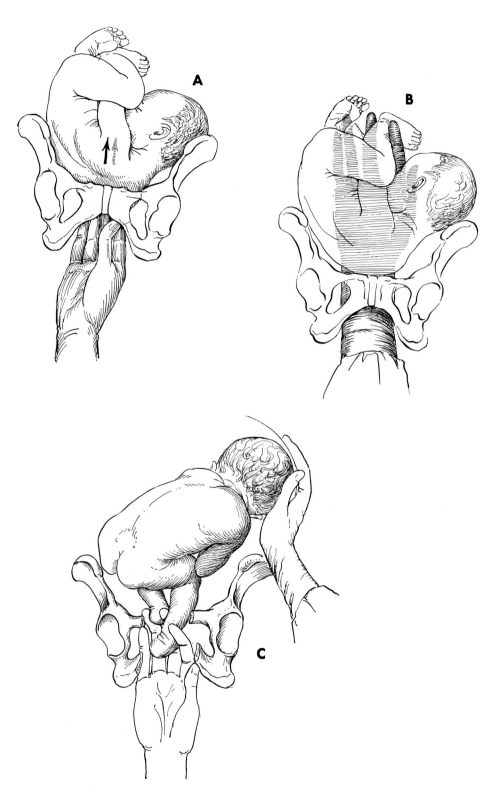

Plate 48

Version in scapula right posterior position

The maneuvers necessary to deliver the infant from a scapula posterior position are similar to, but the reverse of, those used when the shoulder lies anteriorly, but the dangers, preparations, and necessary precautions are identical.

A. The infant's shoulder is disengaged, and it and the body are pushed upward out of the pelvis.

B. The operator's hand is passed upward behind the pubis into the uterus until the feet can be identified.

C. Both feet (or only the posterior foot), are grasped and pulled downward through the anterior part of the pelvis in order to rotate the infant's body until the ventral surface and the feet lie over the pelvic inlet.

Plate 48

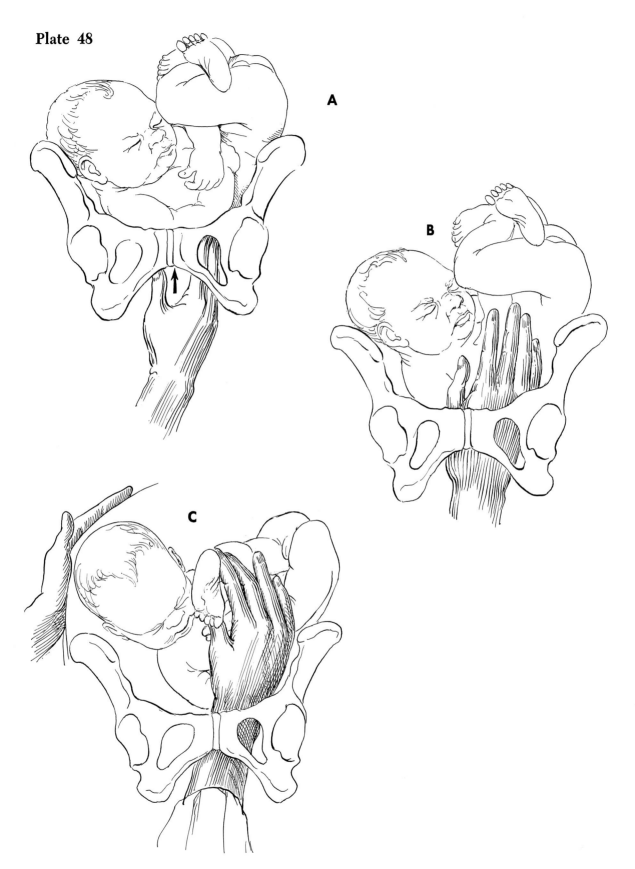

A

B

C

Plate 48 *Concluded*

Version in scapula right posterior position

D. The infant's back is now directed toward the fundus of the uterus; the feet lie in or above the dilated cervix, and the head lies to the right and above the pelvic brim.

E. With further traction, the feet are pulled through the vagina while the buttocks come into the pelvic inlet, and the head rotates upward into the fundus. The extraction is now completed in the usual manner.

Plate 48 *Concluded*

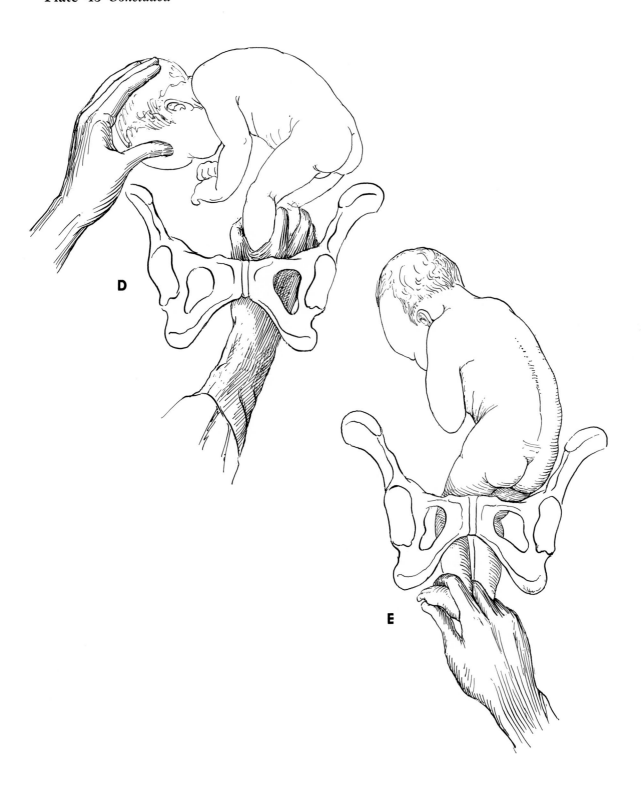

Plate 49

Version in vertex position

Although version and extraction are not often indicated except in transverse lie, in an occasional instance this may be a satisfactory method for completing delivery when the head presents. It is used most often for the delivery of the second of twins and occasionally when the umbilical cord prolapses and delivery by forceps or cesarean section is for some reason not feasible. One of the latter two methods is almost always preferable in the management of prolapsed cord or abnormal positions of the fetus, and for all practical purposes version need be performed only for delivery of the second of twins if intrauterine anoxia develops and the baby cannot be delivered by simple rupture of the membranes or by forceps extraction. It may actually take longer to prepare and anesthetize the patient properly for version than to deliver the baby by some other method. Thus it is not necessarily a rapid method of delivery.

Here, as in the transverse lies, the cervix must be completely dilated, the pelvic size adequate, the amniotic sac intact or the membranes only recently ruptured, and the patient anesthetized until uterine activity is abolished. An intravenous infusion should be started, and the blood should be available. Episiotomy is usually indicated in primigravidas, but it probably will not be necessary until the version has been completed.

A. Sterile vaginal examination is performed to determine the position of the infant and to make certain that the cervix is completely dilated. The head is disengaged and pushed upward out of the pelvis.

B. The operator, wearing an elbow-length version glove well lubricated with green soap, inserts his hand and arm through the cervix, the fingers separating the membranes from the wall of the lower segment until the hand is completely inside the uterine cavity. Great care must be taken to avoid detaching the placenta. The membranes are perforated, the hand and forearm plugging the defect to prevent the escape of too much fluid; the feet are identified, and the umbilical cord is located. If the cord lies between the legs, it is slipped over one foot so that the baby will not be astride it after the version is completed. The maneuvers are most easily carried out if the right hand is used when the ventral surface of the baby is directed toward the left lateral uterine wall and the left hand used when the baby is directed toward the right lateral uterine wall.

Plate 49

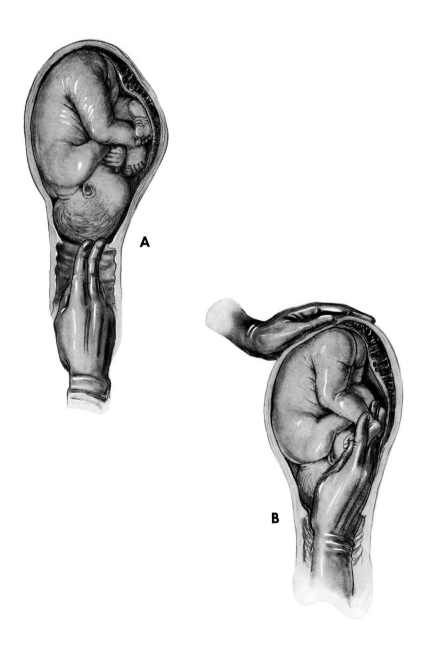

A

B

Plate 49 *Concluded*

Version in vertex position

C. The feet are firmly grasped and pulled downward toward the cervix. The breech, of course, will follow, and at this stage the baby is doubled upon itself and flexion of both the head and the spine is exaggerated. When the buttocks have been pulled downward to about the same level as the head, the head will begin to rise upward toward the fundus. It is not usually necessary to manipulate the head with the hand on the outside, but if it does not rise as the legs are pulled down, it can be pushed upward by pressure through the uterine wall. Pressure should usually not be applied until the buttocks have been pulled down to the level of the vertex.

D. The version is complete, and if the patient has been properly anesthetized and the manipulations properly performed, the head should be flexed and the arms folded across the chest in a normal attitude. The anesthetic can be discontinued during the subsequent extraction of the infant because the need for deep anesthesia is over. This permits the patient to reach a less profound anesthetic level as the baby is being delivered, uterine contractions will recur, and blood loss during the third stage of labor will be reduced.

It is wise to explore the uterus manually in search of an injury after the placenta has been delivered.

242

Plate 49 *Concluded*

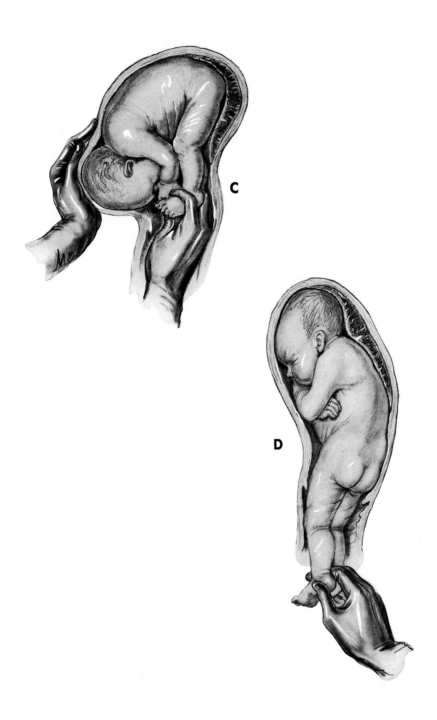

Chapter 12

Cesarean section

In spite of the fact that cesarean section can be performed with a maternal mortality rate no higher than 0.1% to 0.2%, it is not yet as safe as vaginal delivery. Its use, therefore, should be limited to those patients for whom it will be likely to improve the end result without adding to the risk. The incidence with which cesarean section needs to be performed varies with geographic location and from hospital to hospital, but in general at least 5% of pregnancies are terminated by abdominal delivery.

INDICATIONS

Mechanical dystocia. Cesarean section can logically be performed if the size and shape of the bony pelvis will not permit passage of the infant or if the birth canal is occluded by a fibroma, an ovarian neoplasm, or some other tumor. *Abnormalities in pelvic architecture* can usually be recognized early in pregnancy, but the decision to perform cesarean section can only occasionally be made before actual disproportion has been demonstrated by a test of labor. Elective cesarean section for term-sized infants in normal vertex positions can be considered whenever the true conjugate is less than 8 cm. or the bituberous diameter is less than 7 cm., but in either case a short period of labor will do no harm.

Obstructing tumors should usually be removed during early pregnancy, but cesarean section is justifiable if they are first discovered during the last half of pregnancy and cannot be dislodged from the pelvis.

Certain patients with *unverified disproportion* can also be delivered abdominally. For instance, if the membranes rupture spontaneously while the cervix is still long and firm, there may be a latent period of several days before labor begins spontaneously or can be induced. Under these conditions the uterus almost always becomes infected, and the risk is considerably increased if cesarean section because of disproportion eventually becomes necessary. Cesarean section should be performed within

244

twelve to eighteen hours after the membranes rupture when vaginal and x-ray examinations indicate that normal delivery may be impossible and a satisfactory test of labor cannot be given.

Bleeding. Almost all women in whom a diagnosis of *complete placenta previa* is made should be delivered by cesarean section, but those with minor degrees of low implantation, particularly if they are multiparas, can sometimes be delivered vaginally. Cesarean section is more often necessary in primigravidas than in multiparas with minor degrees of placenta previa, but unless the physician can anticipate a short labor in multiparas, abdominal delivery may be preferable; this is particularly true if active bleeding continues.

The mild degrees of *premature placental separation* that usually occur during labor have little influence on maternal and infant mortality, but *complete abruptio placentae* certainly does. Cesarean section is indicated for patients with complete abruptio placentae, even though the baby is already dead, if labor cannot be initiated by rupture of the membranes and oxytocic stimulation. The excessive bleeding accompanying this lesion may be a result of hypofibrinogenemia; hence the clotting mechanism should always be checked when abruptio placentae is suspected. If a clotting defect does develop and cesarean section is selected as the most appropriate method for delivery, the operation should be performed immediately after the defect has been corrected by the administration of blood and fibrinogen. If the procedure is delayed, the fibrinogen will again be utilized and excessive bleeding will occur during the procedure.

Malposition. The fetus in transverse lie or in brow and face positions should be delivered by cesarean section if the malposition cannot be corrected and the prospects for safe vaginal termination do not seem to be good.

Breech positions. Breech position alone does not often warrant abdominal delivery, but cesarean section may be indicated if the pregnancy is of at least thirty-eight weeks' duration and the pelvic measurements are reduced, if the uterine contractions are irregular and ineffective and the labor does not progress satisfactorily, if the membranes rupture prematurely, if the baby weighs at least 2000 grams and labor cannot be initiated within twenty-four hours, if the cord prolapses, or if fetal distress develops during the first stage of labor.

Fetal indications. Cesarean section may occasionally be indicated for *prolapsed cord* or for *cord entanglement* if the baby, as evaluated by fetal heart rate, has not suffered serious anoxia. If the heart rate is constantly slow and irregular, cesarean section is usually contraindicated because the baby is already badly damaged.

In some women, particularly those with chronic vascular renal disease, the *fetus repeatedly dies in utero* during the last four weeks of pregnancy. Cesarean section while the baby is still alive may permit the delivery of a healthy infant who will survive. It may be possible in such patients to assess the condition of the baby by serial determinations of maternal urinary estriol during the last trimester of pregnancy. These determinations may not be completely accurate if maternal renal function is reduced. Repeated late intrauterine death may occasionally occur with severe erythroblastosis. Repeated determinations of the optical density of amniotic fluid during the last trimester will indicate whether or not the baby is affected and the progress of the disease. This will help in selecting a proper time for delivery.

Occasionally *oversized infants* may be injured during vaginal delivery even though the pelvis seems normal. If this has occurred during the patient's past deliveries and the present infant also appears to be large, abdominal delivery may be warranted. Cephalopelvic disproportion may occur if the infant is overdeveloped even though the size of the pelvis is normal.

Medical complications. Women with *diabetes mellitus* should often be delivered several weeks before term, and since it may be difficult to induce labor, cesarean section is frequently indicated. Patients with *reduced pulmonary function* due to the destruction of large volumes of lung tissue by tuberculosis, bronchiectasis and similar lesions, or surgical removal can often be delivered more safely abdominally than through the vagina. Cesarean section is contraindicated for most women with *heart disease* unless prolonged labor from disproportion can be anticipated.

Dysfunctional labor. Cesarean section may be indicated if incoordinate uterine activity cannot be corrected by the administration of oxytocic substances.

Toxemia of pregnancy. Labor can usually be induced successfully in women with severe preeclampsia-eclampsia even though they are several weeks from term; hence, abdominal delivery is not often necessary. Cesarean section is more frequently indicated in patients with severe chronic hypertensive disease, particularly if it is accompanied by an acute superimposed process.

Repeat cesarean sections. The incidence of rupture of the cesarean scar during subsequent pregnancies is not definitely known, but when the scar does separate, the infant may be extruded into the peritoneal cavity where it expires, and bleeding may be profuse. Rupture of an incision in the upper segment of the uterus is usually more disastrous than one in the lower part of the uterus.

Since there is no way of evaluating the integrity and strength of a scar in the uterus and since most ruptures occur during the last week or two of pregnancy or during labor, elective cesarean section late in pregnancy will prevent this complication in many patients. Since the operation is performed in the interests of the infant as well as the mother, little is gained if the mortality from the delivery of premature infants exceeds that of the expected loss from rupture; hence, the physician must be certain by history, palpation, and x-ray examination that the infant is of reasonable size. If the menstrual history is uncertain, the physician may wait until the cervix ripens or even until labor begins before operating. This, however, nullifies the advantage of a planned procedure during which the patient can be fasted and properly prepared.

PREOPERATIVE PREPARATION

Preoperative preparation depends in part upon whether the operation is planned or is an emergency procedure, as so many cesarean sections must be. The risk in the latter is increased because the patient may have eaten recently and may even have some temporary physical abnormality that would be a reason for delaying an elective operation.

The abdomen and perineum are shaved and an enema is administered the night before an elective operation, but the enema is usually omitted in an emergency cesarean. Food and fluid are withheld for twelve hours before an elective operation. Although blood transfusion is not necessary during every abdominal delivery, the blood loss often is excessive, and compatible blood should be available for immediate use.

The medications given the mother cross the placenta to the infant's circulation; consequently, preoperative administration of opiates or barbiturates may depress the infant and interfere with the initiation of respiration after delivery. An adequate sedative effect can be achieved with 50 mg. promazine (Sparine) or 5 to 10 mg. prochlorperazine (Compazine) and 0.4 to 0.6 mg. atropine sulfate about thirty to sixty minutes before the operation is started.

Immediately before the patient is placed in position on the operating table, the bladder is emptied with a rubber catheter that is left in place to provide constant drainage during the procedure. The abdomen is prepared by first cleansing the skin and then applying an antiseptic solution. The area to be prepared includes the upper third of the thighs and the entire anterior portion of the trunk between the pubis and the xyphoid and laterally to the midaxillary line.

ANESTHESIA

Regional anesthesia with single-injection spinal, epidural, or local technics is preferable because such methods have little effect upon the infant as long as the mother's blood pressure remains stable. Inhalation anesthesia, particularly if deep and protracted, may delay the spontaneous initiation of respiration in the baby and in general is less desirable than one of the regional methods; however, cyclopropane and oxygen may be preferable to spinal or epidural anesthesia in women who are bleeding and who are poor candidates for local infiltration.

When cyclopropane is used, it is essential that the infant be delivered

247

as rapidly as possible, because the gas, which crosses the placenta with ease, will anesthetize the infant as well as the mother. This will interfere with the establishment of its own respiratory pattern. The mother is prepared and draped before the anesthetic is started, and the incision is made as soon as pain sensation has been obliterated. It is not necessary to wait for muscle relaxation, as with gynecologic abdominal operations.

POSTOPERATIVE CARE

During the immediate postoperative period, the patient is best cared for in a recovery room where she can be under constant observation until she is conscious and her blood pressure and pulse have become stabilized. If she must be transferred to her own room immediately, she should be checked at least every fifteen minutes during the first few hours.

Sedation. Most women do not have a great deal of pain following cesarean section, but some discomfort is inevitable, particularly during the first twenty-four to forty-eight hours. Discomfort can be kept at a minimum, however, without jeopardizing the patient. The administration of 50 mg. Sparine every six to eight hours for the first forty-eight hours will produce emotional and physical relaxation and will permit smaller dosages of narcotics; 50 mg. Demerol every three hours as needed will usually be adequate when Sparine is used; by the third day, 0.065 Gm. codeine and 0.65 Gm. aspirin every three to four hours usually is sufficient.

If the patient cannot sleep, 0.1 to 0.2 Gm. sodium pentobarbital may be given at bedtime.

Food and fluid. A total of 2500 ml. of fluid is administered intravenously during the day of operation and again the first postoperative day. Thereafter, the average patient can take enough fluid orally to satisfy her needs. Vomiting usually is minimal after cesarean section; consequently, there is little loss of sodium chloride and no need to replace electrolytes. Fluid requirements can be met satisfactorily with 5% dextrose in distilled water. If the patient is dehydrated, has lost a considerable amount of blood, is infected, or has been vomiting, the necessary fluids are determined by her physiologic needs.

A liquid diet can ordinarily be taken on the first postoperative day and a soft diet on the second and third days. Most women can be returned to a full-house diet by the fourth day. If unusual vomiting does occur, it can generally be controlled with 5 to 10 mg. Compazine every six to eight hours.

Ambulation. Most women can get out of bed the day after operation. The patient should first be encouraged to sit on the edge of the bed and then to walk a few steps. She is usually more comfortable if a tight abdominal binder is applied before she attempts to get up. Activity is gradually increased until she is spending much of her day up and about by the end of the week.

Bladder. Most women void without difficulty following cesarean section, and the catheter can usually be removed a few hours after the patient is returned to her room whenever it becomes evident that the kidneys are functioning normally. The patient may be more comfortable, however, if the catheter is left in place until the intravenous fluids have been administered on the first postoperative day.

Bowel. Unless the patient defecates spontaneously, an enema is administered on the morning of the third postoperative day, and milk of magnesia or another cathartic can be ordered daily as needed until the patient is discharged from the hospital.

Plate 50

Lower segment cesarean section

The main advantage of the lower segment operation is that the incision lies beneath the bladder and can be completely excluded from the peritoneal cavity, thereby reducing the incidence of postoperative ileus and adhesion formation. It can be used with relative safety after the membranes have ruptured or after several hours of labor because even though bacteria have invaded the uterus, seepage of uterine contents into the peritoneal cavity is minimal. Rupture of the scar in subsequent pregnancies is generally thought to occur less frequently when the lower segment is opened.

Lower segment operations can be performed in patients who are not yet in labor as well as in those in whom labor is well advanced even though they may be potentially infected. It is quite suitable for most women with placenta previa and abruptio placentae. In general, most cesarean sections should be of the lower segment type.

Local anesthesia. Local anesthesia is quite satisfactory for the performance of cesarean section in many women and is far less dangerous than any of the other anesthetic technics. Of course it does not provide as complete relief from pain, particularly during the extraction of the infant, as do spinal or inhalation methods, but it can be used in at least a third of all cesarean sections if patients are properly selected and prepared. The proposed procedure must be discussed with the patient beforehand in order that she will be aware of what to expect. Women who are unusually fearful and those who tolerate discomfort poorly are not good candidates for local anesthesia.

The administration of 50 to 100 mg. Sparine or 5 to 10 mg. Compazine and 0.4 to 0.6 mg. atropine about one hour preoperatively will relax the patient both physically and emotionally and improve the results of the operation. Either 0.5% lidocaine (Xylocaine) or 0.5% procaine provides satisfactory anesthesia; a total of 150 to 200 ml. of the solution usually is sufficient.

A. A skin wheal is raised in the midline, and the solution is injected subcutaneously with a Pitkin syringe. The solution is injected as the needle is slowly inserted beneath the skin and during its withdrawal. This technic provides a wide anesthetized band on each side of the midline and reduces the possibility of injecting the anesthetic intravenously. It is particularly important to anesthetize the skin and subcutaneous tissue over the ventral surface of the pubis. The skin lateral to the umbilicus is also infiltrated.

250

Plate 50

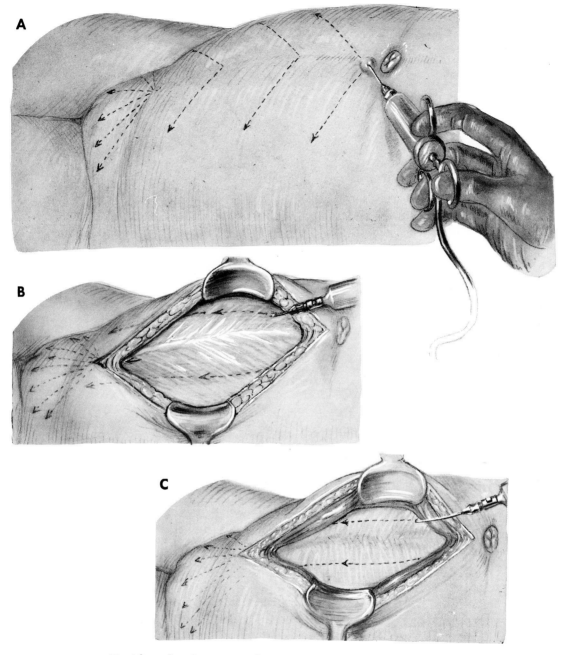

B. After the skin and subcutaneous structures have been incised, the fascia is anesthetized. The terminal branches of the segmental nerves that traverse the abdominal wall can be blocked by linear injections beneath the fascia on each side of the midline. Anesthetic solution is also injected behind the pubis in a fan-shaped pattern.

C. After the fascial incision is made, the properitoneal structures and the peritoneum are anesthetized. It is not necessary to infiltrate the peritoneum simply to cut it, but the pain caused by grasping it with instruments and separating the cut edges will be reduced by the injection.

Plate 51

Lower segment cesarean section

A. The point at which the loose peritoneum overlying the bladder and the lower segment becomes adherent to the uterine wall is identified, and a bleb is raised by injecting 5 to 10 ml. of the anesthetic solution beneath the loose peritoneum.

B. The upper border of the lower segment can be clearly demarcated by massaging the fluid in the bleb laterally with the fingertips. This will indicate the highest level at which the peritoneum can be incised.

Plate 51

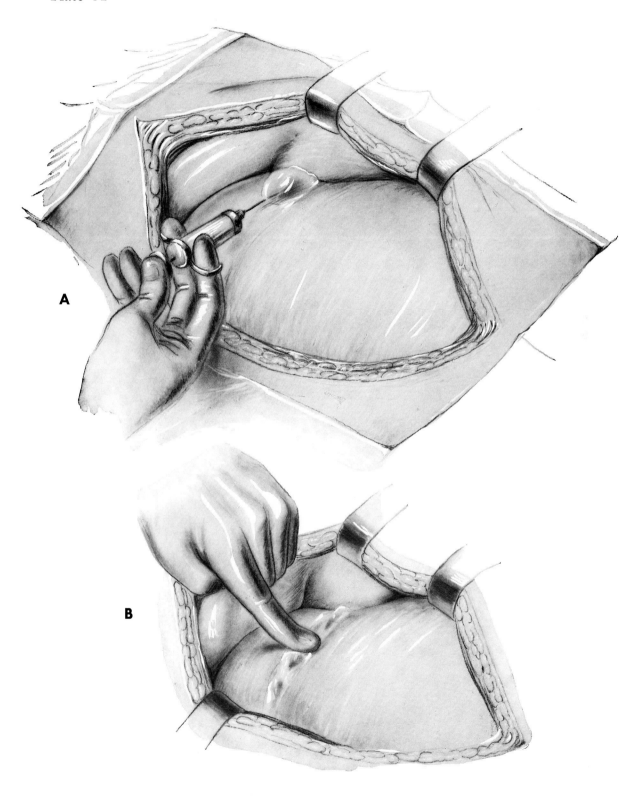

A

B

Plate 51 *Continued*

Lower segment cesarean section

C. The peritoneum is incised along the border of its attachment to the uterine wall between the round ligaments, and the free surface is grasped with clamps and elevated to expose the dome of the bladder and the fibrous tissue by which it is attached to the uterine wall. The fibrous attachments are cut with scissors until a cleavage plane is developed. The bladder is attached most firmly in the midline.

D. After the cleavage plane has been established, the bladder can be stripped downward off the lower segment with ease. This is accomplished by finger dissection or with a folded gauze sponge held by ring forceps. There is little bleeding if the dissection is carried out in the proper plane.

Plate 51 *Continued*

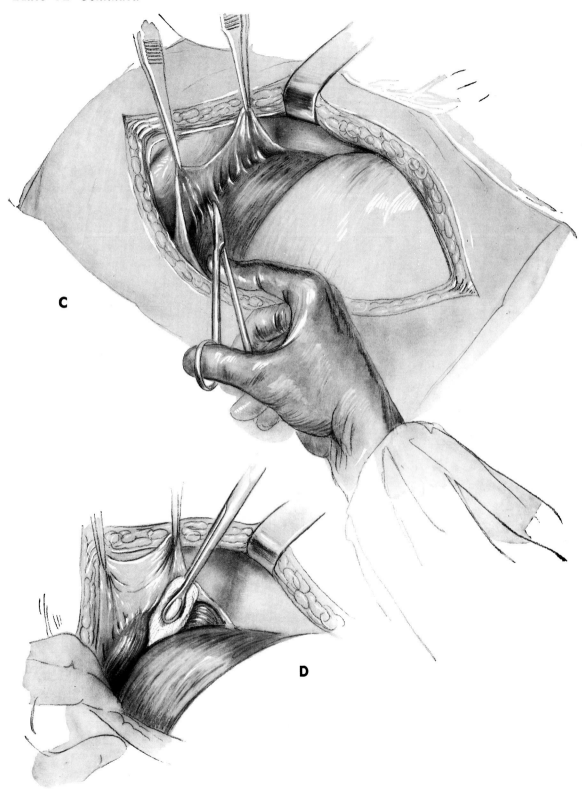

C

D

Plate 51 *Continued*

Lower segment cesarean section

E. The peritoneal edge is sutured to the lower angle of the incision to hold it and the bladder out of the way. A transverse incision is made through the uterine wall about 2 cm. below the junction of the thin passive lower segment and the thick contractile upper segment. The membranes that bulge through the short incision can be perforated now or later when the incision has been completed.

A transverse incision is usually preferable because it can be kept entirely in the thin lower segment. This is particularly true if the lower segment has not been expanded by several hours of labor. If cesarean section is performed after labor has been in progress for some time, the lower segment is usually long enough to permit a longitudinal incision. If an opening of adequate length can be obtained only by carrying the incision into the upper segment, the advantages of the lower segment operation are partially nullified.

F. The bladder is retracted from the field with a DeLee retractor, and the incision is elongated. This can be accomplished by separating the muscle fibers by firm traction at each end of the small opening with the index fingers or by cutting the uterine wall with bandage scissors. There often is less bleeding when the tissue is torn. The incision must be long enough to permit easy extraction of the head.

Plate 51 *Continued*

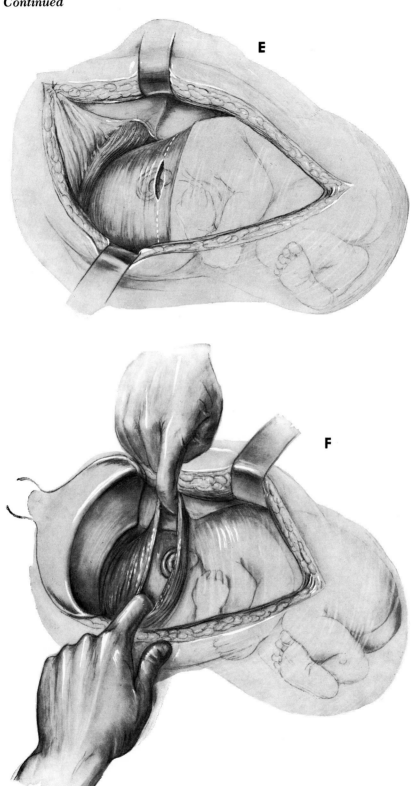

E

F

Plate 51 *Continued*

Lower segment cesarean section

G. The index finger is inserted into the baby's mouth, and the face is rotated anteriorly into the incision.

H. The head has been rotated anteriorly until the entire face lies in the incision, with the chin resting on the uterine wall outside the uterine cavity. The nasopharynx is cleared of amniotic fluid and secretions by suction before the rest of the infant is extracted.

Plate 51 *Continued*

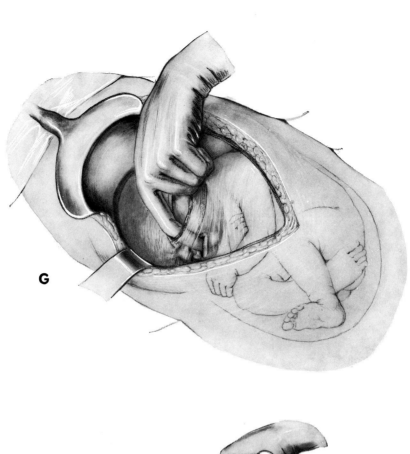

G

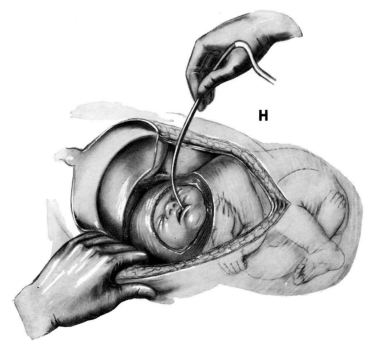

H

Plate 51 *Continued*

Lower segment cesarean section

It is important that the face be exposed and the head delivered with as little force as possible. If the extraction of the head is delayed or difficult, requiring unusual manipulation, the infant may begin to breathe and aspirate large amounts of amniotic fluid and debris. Extraction is facilitated by an adequate incision; if the opening seems too small, it should be enlarged at once.

If the patient has been in labor many hours, the infant's head has usually been elongated by molding and a large caput has formed. Under these circumstances it may be difficult to extract the head because it is wedged in the upper part of the pelvis. Extraction will be easier if the head is dislodged by an assistant who pushes upward on the presenting part through the vagina. Of course, this must be done with all sterile precautions.

I. A single forceps blade can be used as a vectis to pry the head through the incision. The blade is slid between the infant's cheek and the uterine wall until it lies with its cephalic curve applied to the side of the head.

J. The blade is then manipulated around the head until it lies over the occipital area.

Plate 51 *Continued*

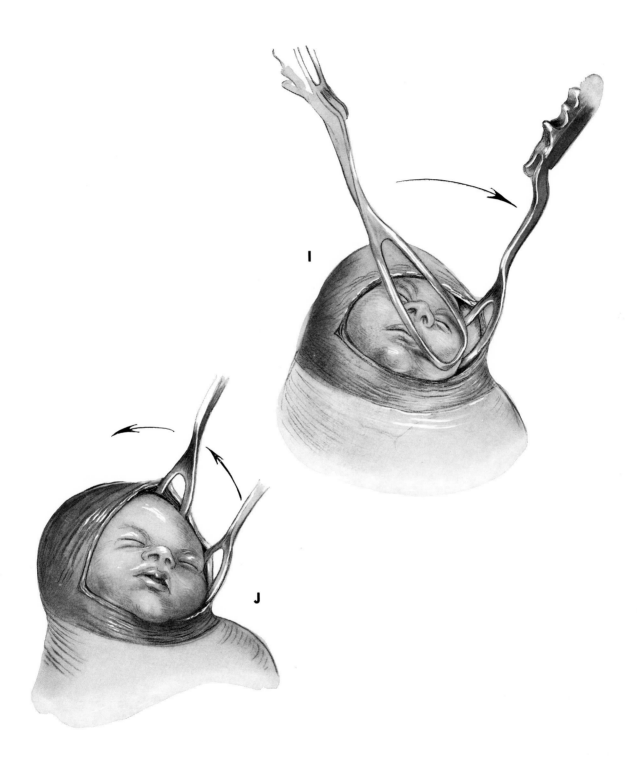

Plate 51 *Continued*

Lower segment cesarean section

K. The head is delivered through the incision by upward pressure with the forceps blade.

L. An alternative method for delivering the head is to extract it with forceps after the face has been rotated into the incision. The forceps blades are applied on the lateral sides of the head in the mento-occipital diameter, with the anterior surface of the instrument directed toward the pubis. The head is extended and the chin is pulled upward until it is completely free, after which the forceps handles are depressed toward the mother's abdominal wall as traction is applied; this tends to flex the head and pull it through the opening.

Plate 51 *Continued*

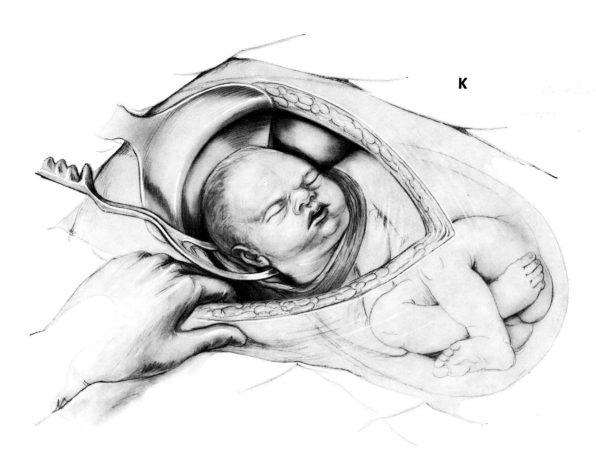

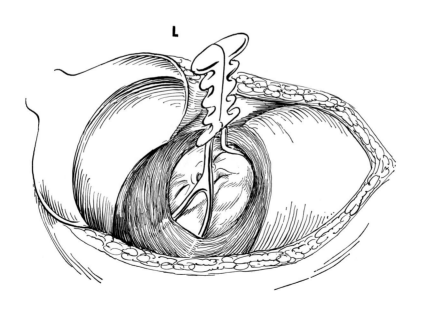

Plate 51 *Continued*

Lower segment cesarean section

    M. The head is grasped in both hands and pulled upward until the posterior shoulder and axilla can be seen emerging from the uterine cavity.

    N. The head is supported in the left hand while the anterior shoulder is pulled farther downward by traction with the index finger. The remainder of the extraction of the baby should be slow and deliberate to permit the uterine muscle fibers to retract gradually as the uterus is emptied.

Plate 51 *Continued*

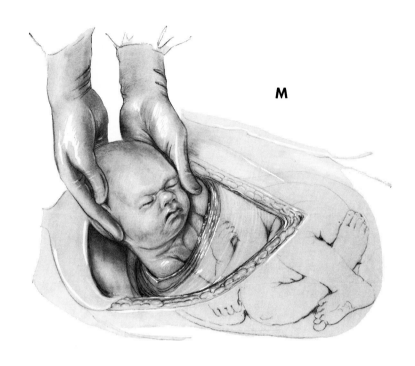

M

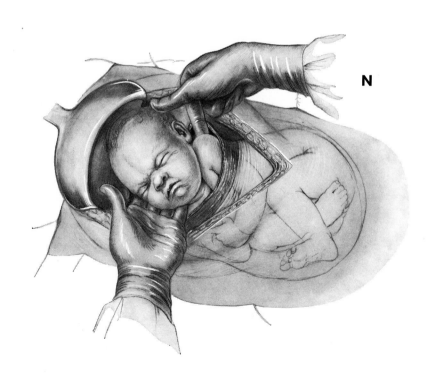

N

Plate 51 *Continued*

Lower segment cesarean section

O. The posterior shoulder is brought completely through the incision by traction in the axilla. At this stage of the operation it often is helpful to remove the wound retractors, which may be in the way.

P. The baby is slowly extracted from the uterus by traction in the axillae. There should be no difficulty in removing the body once the head and shoulders are free.

Plate 51 *Continued*

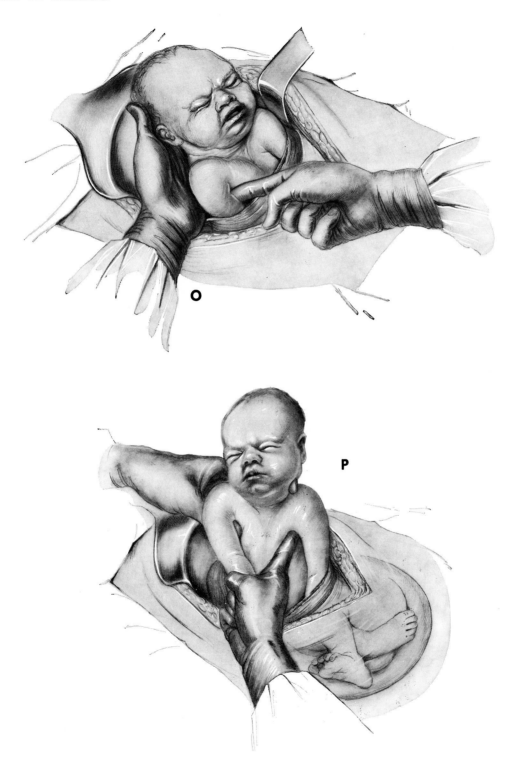

O

P

Plate 51 *Continued*

Lower segment cesarean section

Q. The infant is placed on the mother's abdomen or thighs until the cord is cut. Here, as in vaginal delivery, the cord is milked several times from the placenta toward the infant to infuse the infant with blood that might otherwise be discarded with the placenta. The cord is not milked in infants who may have erythroblastosis fetalis. The cord is then doubly clamped and cut, and the infant is placed in a heated crib under the care of a physician or an experienced nursery nurse. It is helpful to have a physician in attendance whose only responsibility is the care of the infant. The operator can then devote his entire attention to the mother whether or not the baby is doing well.

The placenta is still in the upper segment of the uterus, although it may by now be partially detached. The walls of the lower segment are flaccid, and unless there is considerable bleeding, the internal os can be identified through the fetal membranes covering it. Excessive bleeding from sinuses at the edges of the incision can be controlled with Allis clamps or similar instruments.

Plate 51 *Continued*

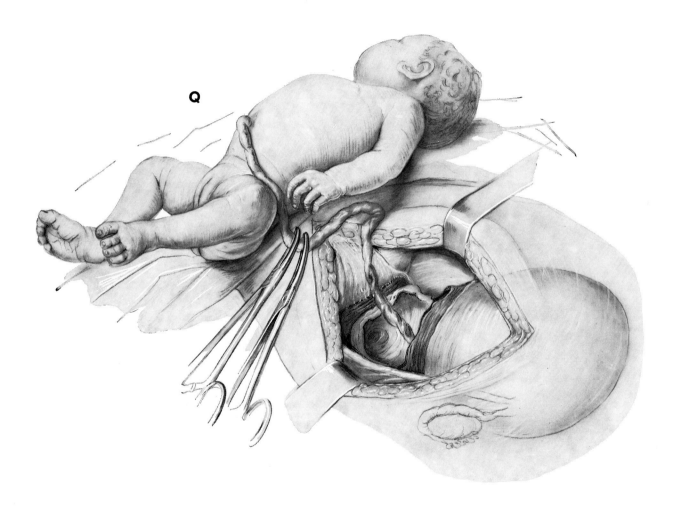

Q

Plate 51 *Continued*

Lower segment cesarean section

R. If the placenta has not already separated from the uterine wall, it can be detached by manual manipulation. The operator's fingers, with the palmar surface upward, are insinuated between the maternal surface of the placenta and the uterine wall until it is completely free.

S. The hand is turned over in order that it may seize the placenta and deliver it from the cavity. The operator uses the other hand to aid in the extraction.

It often is preferable to wait a few moments until the uterus contracts and separates the placenta spontaneously. This will reduce the blood loss; while the placenta remains attached and the uterus is quiescent, there will be no bleeding from the placental site. If the placenta is removed and the uterus fails to contract promptly, blood loss from the choriodecidual sinuses may be excessive. The uterus is much less active during and immediately after elective cesarean sections than in those done after a period of labor. Consequently, blood loss from the placental site is likely to be greater in the former.

Plate 51 *Continued*

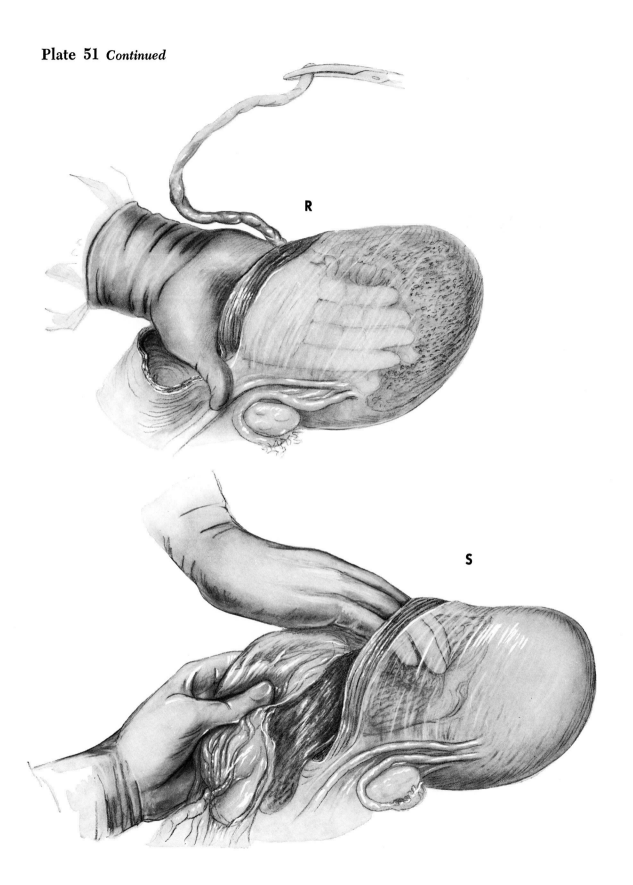

R

S

Plate 51 *Continued*

Lower segment cesarean section

T. The placenta is held in the left hand and elevated until the membranes covering the lower uterine segment are put on a stretch. They usually can be peeled off the uterine wall with little effort; however, if they are unusually adherent or tear, it may be necessary to grasp them with a hemostat.

Any membrane left in this area may occlude the cervical opening and prevent adequate drainage of the uterine contents.

After the placenta has been removed, a uterotonic agent is given to stimulate the uterus to contract. Ergonovine (Ergotrate), 0.2 mg., methylergonovine (Methergine), 0.2 mg., or oxytocin, 1 unit, may be given intravenously by the anesthetist. The oxytocic agent may also be injected directly into the uterine muscle by the surgeon, but there is no advantage to this technic since the drug must be transported through the blood vessels from the injection site to the rest of the uterus.

Plate 51 *Continued*

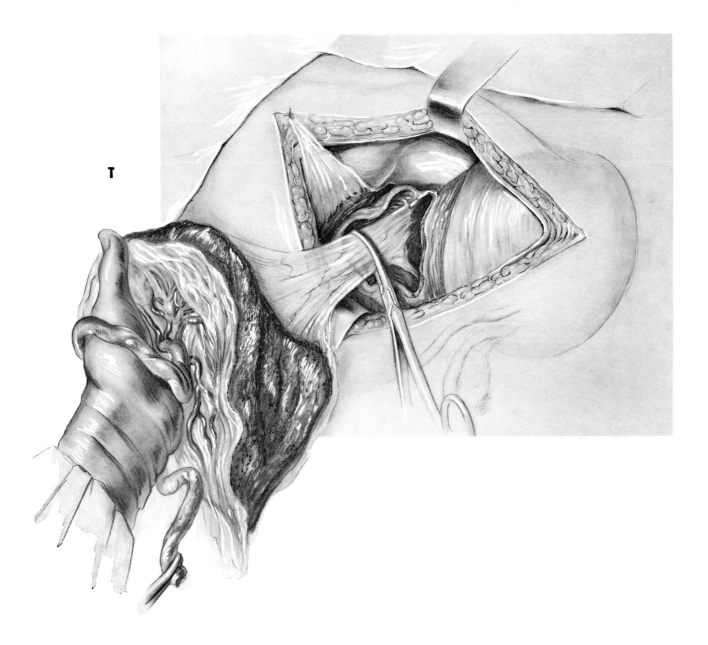

T

Plate 51 *Continued*

Lower segment cesarean section

If cesarean section is performed before labor begins, the cervix is often closed and firm, and drainage may be inadequate. Under such circumstances, it is well to pack the cervix to make certain that it will open and provide an exit for the blood and debris that will collect within the uterine cavity. This is not necessary if the patient has been in labor and the cervix is partially open.

U. A small amount of 2-inch gauze packing is forced into the upper segment, but no attempt is made to pack it tightly.

274

Plate 51 *Continued*

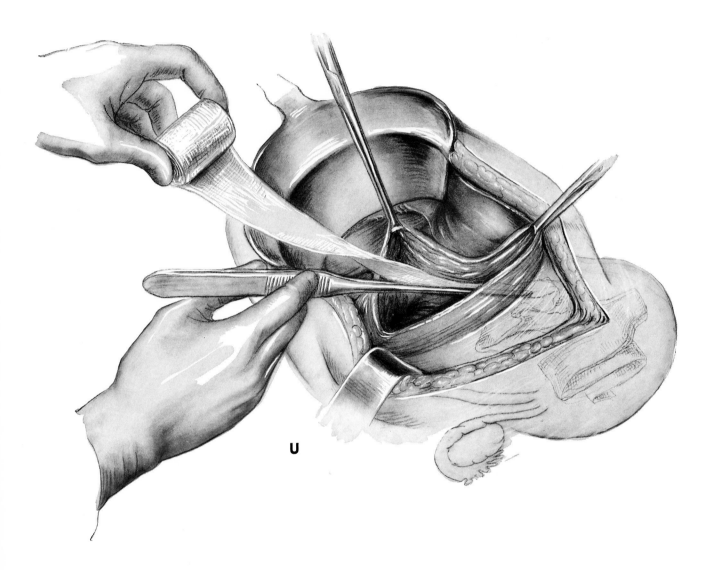

U

Plate 51 *Continued*

Lower segment cesarean section

V. The end of the pack is pushed through the cervix into the vagina. Since it must be removed from below, at least 8 to 10 inches of the pack should be forced into the vagina so that it can be easily identified and seized. The instrument used is discarded because it has passed through the cervix into the unsterile vagina.

The pack is removed by traction from below eight to twelve hours after completion of the operation.

Plate 51 *Continued*

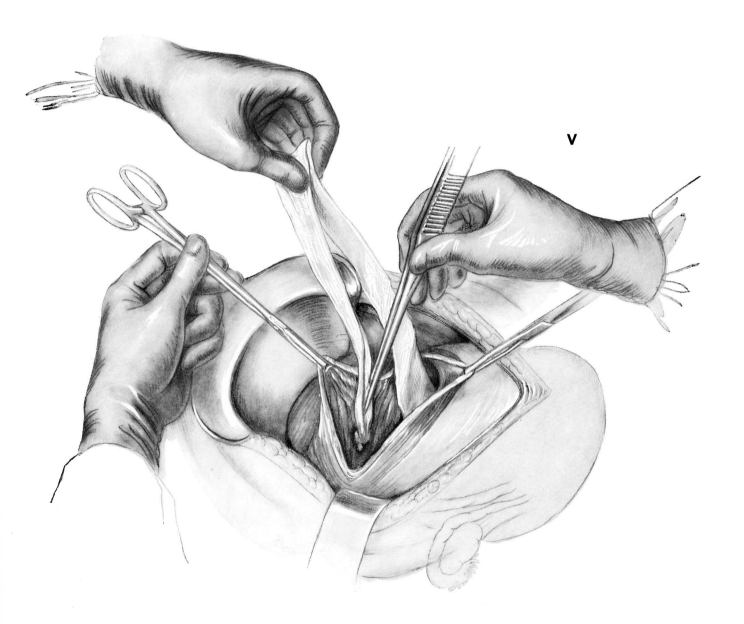

V

Plate 51 *Concluded*

Lower segment cesarean section–closure

The operator can usually close a lower segment incision more easily and accurately than one in the upper part of the uterus because the wall is thin and bleeding usually is less profuse. Careful hemostasis and coaptation of the wound edges reduce the leakage of uterine contents and promote firm healing. This is particularly important if future pregnancies are anticipated. Chromic 0 and 00 catgut is quite adequate for the closure.

W. The first layer of sutures is interrupted and includes the entire thickness of the lower uterine segment. The sutures are placed about 1 cm. apart.

X. The first layer is reinforced with a continuous Lembert stitch that approximates the muscle of the flaccid lower segment over the interrupted sutures.

After all bleeding has been controlled, the wound is extraperitonealized by approximating the cut edges of the peritoneum with a continuous suture of chromic 00 catgut. If a long flap is available, the edges can be overlapped.

The tubes and ovaries should be inspected before the abdominal wall is closed.

Plate 51 *Concluded*

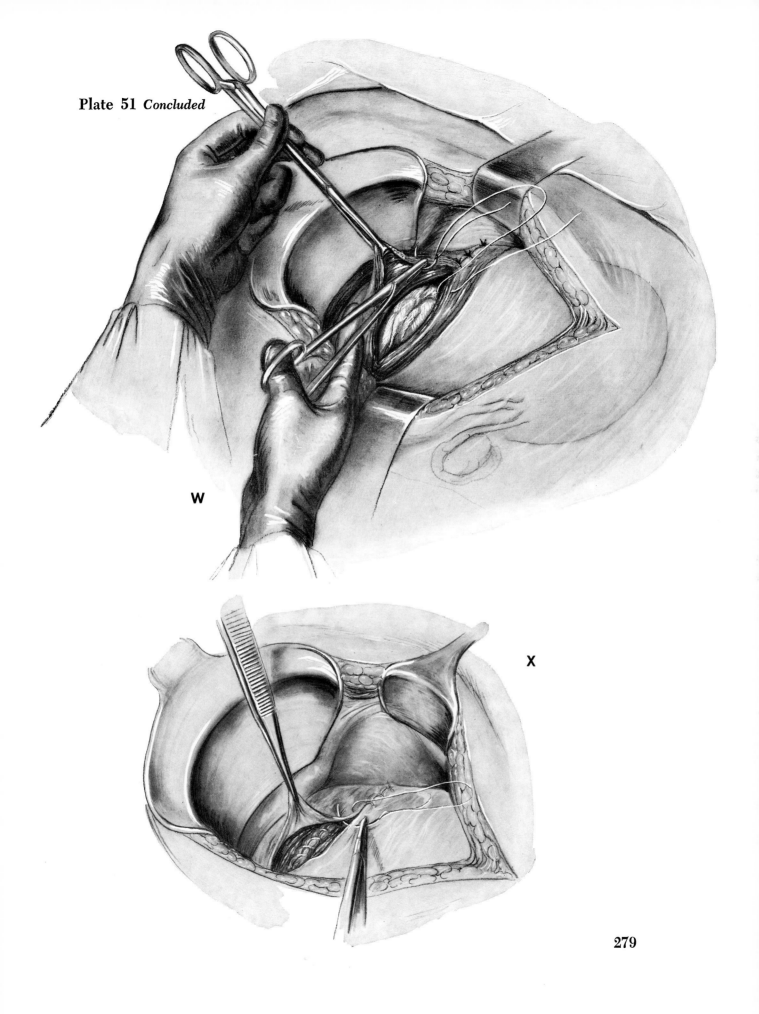

W

X

Plate 52

Classic cesarean section

The ease and rapidity with which classic cesarean section can be performed are offset by the facts that bleeding from the thick upper segment of the uterus is more profuse than from the lower segment and that it tends to heal less well. Most authorities believe that upper segment scars are more prone to rupture during subsequent pregnancies than are those in the lower segment. In addition, rupture of an upper segment scar is likely to be more disastrous than separation of an incision in the lower segment. When an upper segment scar ruptures, the infant is almost always lost because it is extruded into the peritoneal cavity, whereas when a lower segment scar ruptures, the infant usually remains within the uterus. Ileus occurs more frequently and leakage of uterine contents into the peritoneal cavity is more likely to occur than with lower segment operations; consequently, classic section is generally contraindicated after six or more hours of labor and in women in whom the membranes have been ruptured for some time.

The upper segment operation can be performed with reasonable safety as an elective procedure in women who will not become pregnant again, and many operators prefer it for the delivery of women with complete placenta previa. It also is valuable when it is necessary to extract the baby rapidly. Its most important use, however, is for the delivery of infants in transverse presentation with the back down. Extraction through a lower segment incision under these circumstances is difficult and often injurious to the baby.

A. The incision in the abdominal wall can be placed either on the midline between the umbilicus and the pubis or, as is shown here, in the paraumbilical area. For transverse presentation with the ventral surface of the infant directed upward, a high incision permits extraction with less manipulation, but an incision below the umbilicus is usually satisfactory.

B. The uterine wall is exposed, and a small incision is made with a scalpel. The incision is placed as close to the midline as possible because the area is less vascular. If there is considerable dextrorotation of the uterus, it is corrected before the incision is made. The initial incision is extended to the desired length with bandage scissors.

Plate 52

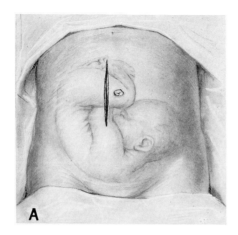

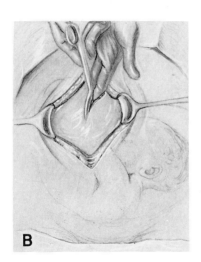

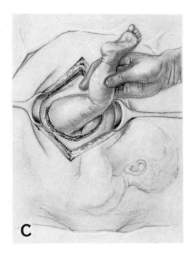

C. The anterior foot of the infant is located and pulled through the uterine incision, and the baby is delivered by maneuvers similar to those used for breech extraction. Delivery of the head can be delayed for a considerable period of time by an incision that is too short.

If the placenta is normally implanted on the anterior wall, it may be cut as the uterus is incised; this will result in bleeding from the placental circulation. The infant's blood loss can be minimized by separating the placenta until the edge can be seen, rupturing the membranes, and pulling out and clamping a loop of umbilical cord.

Plate 52 *Concluded*

Classic cesarean section

After the infant has been delivered, the placenta is extracted manually, and an oxytocic (usually 0.2 mg. Methergine) is injected intravenously to encourage muscle contraction. If the cervix is closed, a pack is pushed down through it into the vagina, the upper portion remaining in the fundus, as described for lower segment operations.

It is more difficult to close the thick contracted muscle wall of the upper segment than the relatively relaxed and thin lower segment, but accurate coaptation of the wound edges and control of bleeding will aid in healing and the development of a strong scar. Chromic 0 catgut on a large full-curved atraumatic needle is quite adequate except for the serosal layer.

D. The first layer of chromic 0 catgut sutures is interrupted and approximates the inner third of the uterine incision. These sutures usually are placed above the decidua, but no harm will result from placing an occasional suture within the uterine cavity.

E. The sutures in the second row are either interrupted or continuous, depending upon the ease with which the wound edges can be approximated and the amount of bleeding. Interrupted sutures are preferable if there is considerable tension, but a continuous stitch provides better hemostasis. A third layer may be necessary if the wall is unusually thick.

F. The serosal suture is continuous. A Lembert suture may be used to advantage.

Plate 52 *Concluded*

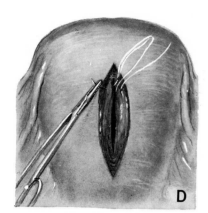

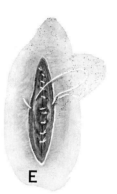

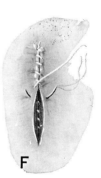

Plate 53

Waters' extraperitoneal cesarean section

The proper application of the available refinements in the management of abnormal labor and the use of the potent antimicrobial agents should eliminate the need for the extraperitoneal operation, because in almost every instance a decision to perform cesarean section can be made before the uterus is infected. However, an occasional patient with intrauterine infection will require cesarean section. Many such patients can be delivered safely by a transperitoneal lower segment procedure during which the infected uterine contents spill into the peritoneal cavity only while the infant is being extracted. The spill can be almost eliminated by the use of gauze packs. The incision is extraperitonealized when the bladder flap is reattached, and subsequent drainage is minimal. Even though the peritoneum will usually inhibit the growth of organisms introduced during the performance of lower segment cesarean section, it does not always respond adequately, and some lethal bacteria are insensitive to the antimicrobial agents now available. Extraperitoneal operations, when properly performed, undoubtedly reduce the risk and should be considered whenever a patient whose uterine cavity is grossly infected must be delivered abdominally. Extraperitoneal operations are somewhat more difficult to perform, and the bladder and ureters are injured more often than during the transperitoneal procedures, but anyone qualified to perform cesarean section can learn the technic. Although there are several methods of performing extraperitoneal cesarean section, I prefer the method developed by Waters, which will be described.

Since a good bit of manipulation is required to expose the lower segment, local infiltration usually does not provide adequate pain relief, and epidural, spinal, or general anesthesia is preferable.

Preparation. An indwelling catheter is inserted into the bladder and connected to a Kelly bottle filled with sterile water stained with methylene blue. The Kelly bottle is elevated on an intravenous standard to a height that will permit the fluid to flow into the bladder when the clamp on the tubing is released. The bladder can be emptied by lowering the Kelly bottle below the level of the operating table.

Plate 53

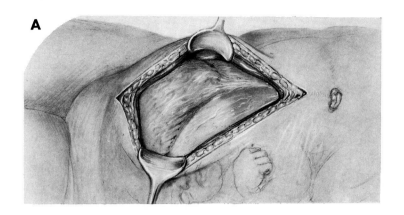

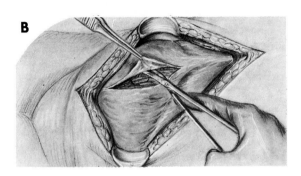

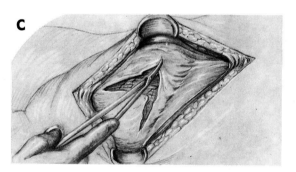

A. The abdominal wall is opened by a left paramedian incision through the skin, subcutaneous tissues, rectus fascia, and muscle. A transverse Cherney incision also provides excellent exposure of the bladder and lower uterine segment. The bladder is then distended with 200 to 250 ml. of the fluid stained with methylene blue to delineate its upper border and the parietovesical fold of the peritoneum.

B. A longitudinal incision is made through the transversalis and perivesical fasciae over the anterior wall of the distended bladder. The operator must take care not to carry the superior end of the incision so high that the anterior fold of the peritoneum that comes down over the bladder will be opened. It is important that the incision be deep enough to expose the vesicle wall, which can be recognized by the blood vessels coursing through the bladder muscularis. The fasciae are bluntly dissected from the bladder on each side of the incision.

C. The fascial layers are then cut transversely, converting the incision into a T-shaped opening through which the distended bladder will bulge.

Plate 53 *Concluded*

Waters' extraperitoneal cesarean section

D. The fascia is pulled superiorly with Allis forceps, and the bladder is gently dissected from the parietovesical peritoneal fold. This is best accomplished by blunt dissection with the fingers or a knife handle rather than with a sharp instrument. The urachus can be isolated, ligated, and incised. The bladder is emptied.

E. The dissection is continued over the left superior surface of the bladder until the vesicouterine fold of peritoneum is exposed. The areolar tissue at the lateral attachment of the fold is relatively loose and can be dissected bluntly until the operator can insinuate his fingers beneath the peritoneal plica. The perivesical fascia lies below the peritoneal fold and between the bladder and the lower uterine segment.

F. A small incision is made in the perivesical fascia, and it is separated from its attachment to the uterine wall by blunt finger dissection. The perivesical fascia is incised transversely below the peritoneal fold until the lower segment is well exposed.

G. The bladder is drawn downward and the right and held out of the field with a broad retractor. Since there is somewhat less uterine area exposed than with a transperitoneal lower segment operation, a transverse crescentic or V-shaped incision in the uterus will provide the most room for delivery of the infant.

The uterine incision is closed in two layers, and the T-shaped opening in the perivesical fascia is closed in one layer. Waters suggests draining the retrovesical space with a soft rubber drain, but I have not found this to be necessary if bleeding in the area can be controlled completely.

Plate 53 *Concluded*

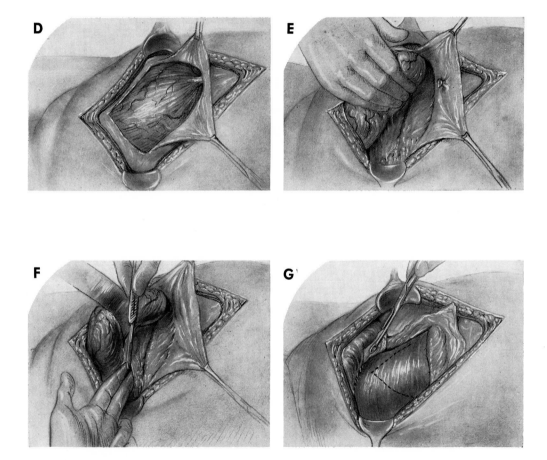

Plate 54

Cesarean hysterectomy

Hysterectomy can be performed in conjunction with cesarean section whenever there is a logical reason for removing the uterus. It is most frequently indicated in multiparas with multiple myomas, but it may also be necessary for the control of hemorrhage from partial rupture of the uterus or from the placental site in the lower uterine segment. Bleeding associated with uteroplacental apoplexy is usually the result of a clotting defect and can be checked by administering fibrinogen; however, if this is ineffectual, hysterectomy may be justifiable. Cesarean hysterectomy may also be chosen for the occasional patient in whom a definite and unequivocable diagnosis of carcinoma in situ of the cervix has been made. It may be much safer to remove the uterus than to perform a transperitoneal or even an extraperitoneal operation in the presence of serious infection such as that which may develop after prolonged obstructed labor.

The general succulence of the tissues makes the planes quite obvious, and the dissection is usually easier than in nonpregnant women. Blood loss usually is greater than with cesarean section alone because of the remarkable hypertrophy of the pelvic blood vessels during pregnancy. Total hysterectomy can be performed without difficulty and is preferable to the subtotal operation unless the additional dissection will prolong the operating time too much in patients who are poor operative risks at best. The baby may be delivered through an incision in either the upper or the lower segment; the incision usually is closed with a continuous stitch of chromic catgut or with wide clamps to control bleeding from the edges during the rest of the operation. Normal ovaries are left in place.

A. The tubes, ovarian ligaments, and round ligaments have been doubly clamped and cut and the stumps ligated, and the dissection is continued downward through the broad ligament. This area usually is more vascular than in nonpregnant women, and it is safer to clamp the tissue before cutting and to place sutures behind the distal clamp. The bladder has already been mobilized to permit delivery of the baby.

B. The peritoneum of the posterior leaf of the broad ligament is incised until the uterine vessels are exposed. These are clamped and severed and the cut ends doubly ligated with chromic 0 catgut. The clamps are placed close to the uterus to avoid the ureters. The ureters can usually be identified easily because of the physiologic dilation of pregnancy.

Plate 54

A

B

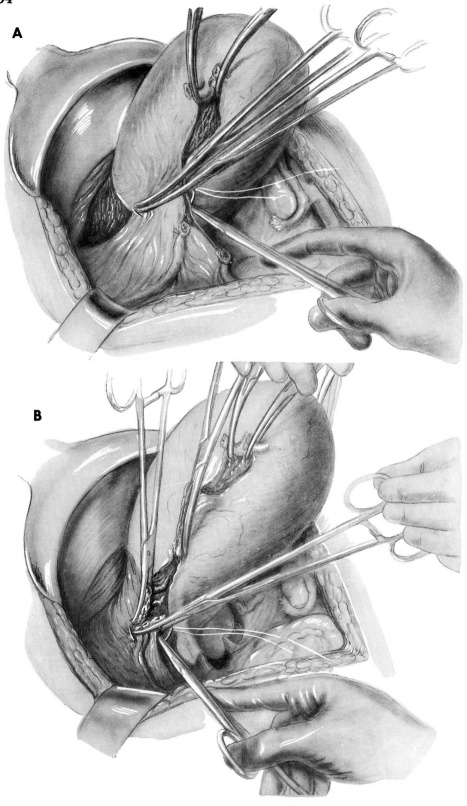

Plate 54 *Continued*

Cesarean hysterectomy

C. The bladder is pushed downward with a gauze sponge until it has been freed from the cervix and upper vagina. The cardinal ligaments and paracervical tissues are clamped, cut, and ligated.

D. The cervix can be removed in several ways, but one of the easiest ways is shown here. A longitudinal incision is made with a knife through the anterior cervix and into the vagina.

Plate 54 *Continued*

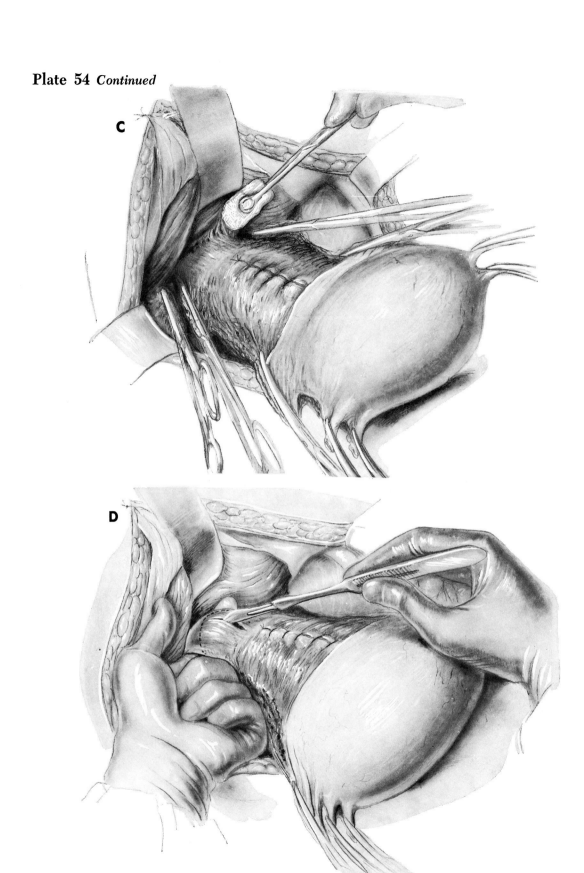

Plate 54 *Continued*

Cesarean hysterectomy

E. The severed anterior cervical lips and the anterior vaginal wall are seized with Allis clamps or Kocher forceps, and the vaginal dissection is begun. The vagina is cut as close to the cervix as possible to maintain a maximum length.

F. The dissection is continued laterally around the cervix toward the uterosacral ligaments. Bleeding areas on the cut edge are controlled with forceps that are not shown here. The uterosacral ligament and the vaginal wall are grasped with Kocher forceps and severed from their attachments to the cervix.

Plate 54 *Continued*

E

F

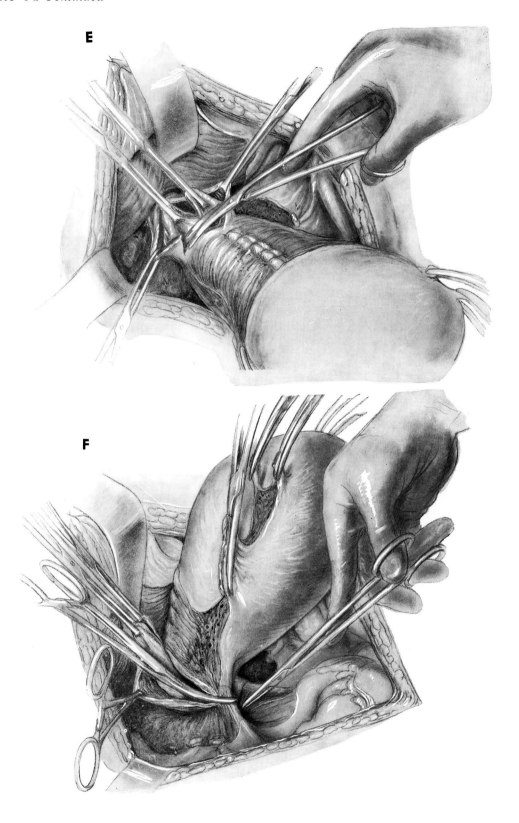

Plate 54 *Continued*

Cesarean hysterectomy

G. The uterosacral ligament is sutured to the vaginal wall with a single suture of chromic 0 catgut. This controls bleeding and anchors it in place.

The peritoneum between the uterosacral ligaments is incised, and the peritoneum and the rectosigmoid are pushed downward slightly when the latter is attached high enough so that it might be injured during the dissection or included in the sutures that will be placed subsequently. The posterior vagina and the opposite uterosacral ligament are incised, and the latter is sutured to the vaginal wall as was the one on the opposite side.

Plate 54 *Continued*

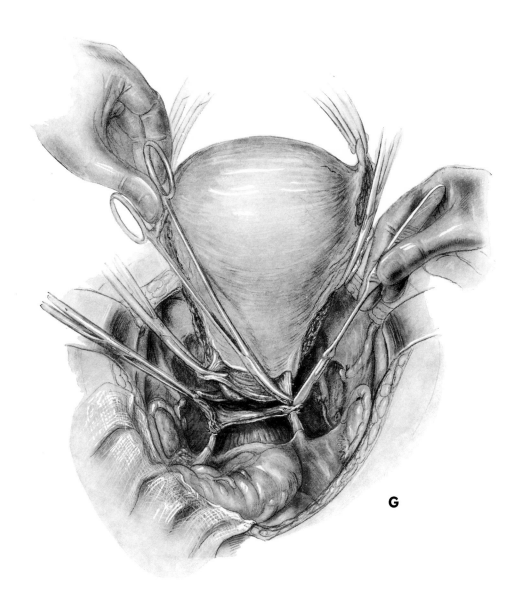

G

Plate 54 *Concluded*

Cesarean hysterectomy

H. The dissection of the vagina has been completed and the uterus and cervix removed. The uterosacral ligaments have already been attached to the cut edge of the vagina, but the cardinal ligaments still lie free. The latter are sutured to each lateral angle of the vagina with an interrupted suture that also serves to control bleeding that may arise from open vessels in the area. The cardinal ligaments provide additional support for the vault of the vagina.

I. The anterior and posterior edges of the vagina are approximated with a continuous suture of chromic catgut. One must make certain that the vaginal mucosa as well as the submucosal tissues are included. If bleeding from the edges is troublesome, a continuous lock stitch or interrupted mattress sutures will provide adequate hemostasis. *Inset.* The cut edge of the bladder peritoneum is sutured to the peritoneum of the posterior pelvis, completely obliterating the raw area.

Plate 54 *Concluded*

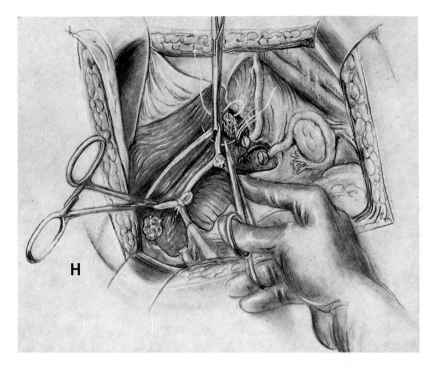

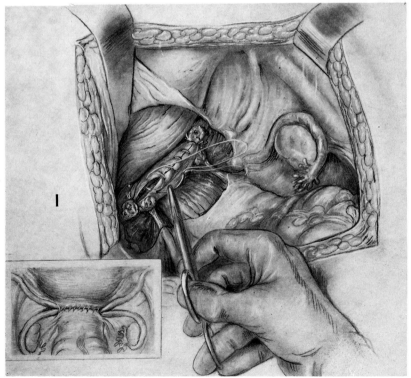

Chapter 13

Placenta previa

DIAGNOSIS

Placenta previa should be suspected as a cause of bleeding that begins during the last few weeks of pregnancy, particularly if the blood is bright red and there is no associated pain. The first bleeding usually appears between the thirtieth and thirty-fourth week and is slight in amount, often consisting only of spotting. Characteristically, the blood loss increases with subsequent episodes of activity; the most serious hemorrhages are precipitated by placental separation during coitus or douching or as a result of digital examination. Since it is impossible by history alone to differentiate placenta previa from less serious conditions that also produce painless bleeding, a planned program of study should be established for the investigation of women who bleed during late pregnancy.

Abdominal palpation. If the placenta is implanted in the lower uterine segment, the presenting part is almost always displaced upward and away from the bulky placenta. For instance, if the implantation site is in the left posterior portion of the uterus, the head will be pushed upward and toward the right anterior quadrant of the pelvis, where it may even override the brim. If a considerable bulk of placenta lies in the pelvic cavity, it will be impossible to force the head through the inlet.

Abnormal presentations occur frequently as a result of placenta previa. Oblique and transverse lies are common. In fact, placenta previa, often of the complete variety, can be diagnosed in about one third of the patients with transverse lie. Because of this possibility, the physician should never perform in his office a rectal or vaginal examination on women with transverse or oblique presentation.

The position of the so-called placental souffle is of little help in locating

298

the implantation site because the physician often is hearing the blood coursing through the uterine vessels on the lateral surface of the uterus rather than through the placental sinuses.

Cervical inspection. The cervix should be inspected to eliminate local lesions as a cause for bleeding. This can be done in the physician's office if proper precautions are used. The external genitalia and the introitus are cleansed with soap and water or a hexachlorophene preparation, and the cervix is exposed with a sterile speculum. The physician may wipe the portio vaginalis cervicis clean with a sterile cotton ball, but he should never insert an instrument or an examining finger into the cervical canal.

The possibility of placenta previa cannot be dismissed simply because a source of bleeding is discovered on the cervix; this is particularly true if blood can be seen coming from the canal. Bleeding cervical lesions should be studied further by cytologic examination and biopsy.

X-ray placentography. It often is possible to locate the placental site by x-ray study, using the soft tissue technic. Three exposures are made: an anteroposterior, a standing lateral through the body of the uterus, and a standing lateral through the pelvis.

Placenta previa can be eliminated if the placental shadow is located in the upper segment. The diagnosis is often made by exclusion; if the placental shadow cannot be identified in the upper segment, and if the presenting part is elevated above the pelvic brim and displaced from the center of the inlet, the placenta is likely to be implanted in the lower part of the uterus. Even though the diagnosis is made by x-ray study, the physician can determine the extent of the lesion only by actually palpating the interior of the uterus.

Radioisotopic scanning. The placental site can be located accurately by using a material such as activated iodinated human serum albumin (RISA). The albumin is injected intravenously and is disseminated throughout the entire maternal circulatory system. Since there is a large volume of blood moving slowly through the choriodecidual space, the amount of activated material will be greater in this area than in the rest of the uterus. The area over which the placenta is attached can be delineated with considerable accuracy by checking each of twelve areas over the anterior surface of the uterus with a scintillation counter. Since the activated albumin is concentrated at the placental site, the counts will be higher over that area than over the rest of the uterus.

This method is at least as accurate as x-ray localization during the last ten weeks of pregnancy, and more accurate earlier; it subjects both the mother and the baby to less radiation than do conventional methods. It is less accurate than x-ray examination if the placenta is attached posteriorly.

Vaginal examination. It is necessary to perform vaginal examination at some time in any patient suspected of having placenta previa because the physician can make a definite diagnosis and establish a plan for treatment only after he knows the extent of cervical effacement and dilation and how much of the opening is covered by placental tissue. Unfortunately, the manipulations necessary to determine the condition of the cervix and to feel the placenta usually will separate more of the placenta from the uterine wall and increase the blood loss; in fact, severe hemorrhage is sometimes precipitated by even the most gentle vaginal or rectal examination.

Because of the possibility of an overwhelming hemorrhage, vaginal examination of patients who are bleeding during the last few weeks of pregnancy should be performed only in the operating room after blood has been made available for transfusion, instruments have been prepared for cesarean section, and the operating team has been assembled. If bleeding is increased considerably by the examination or if abdominal delivery is thought to be preferable to vaginal termination, the physician can perform cesarean section immediately.

Usually vaginal examination should be performed at once if the pregnancy is of at least thirty-seven weeks' duration even though the bleeding is scant or at any stage of gestation if the bleeding is profuse. If bleeding is slight and the pregnancy is of less than thirty-six weeks' duration, vaginal examination should usually be delayed until it becomes necessary because of the possibility of hemorrhage or until the pregnancy has advanced beyond thirty-seven weeks, because the manipulation may produce bleeding that can be controlled only by delivery of an infant too premature to survive. An attempt should be made to identify the placental implantation site by x-ray examination or radioisotopic scanning studies.

The examination is performed with the patient in lithotomy position. It is not necessary to administer an anesthetic unless the patient is unusually apprehensive. After the examiner has scrubbed and has donned sterile gloves, he prepares the vulva as he would for delivery and carefully inserts his fingers into the vagina. He first palpates around the cervix in the fornices in an attempt to detect placental tissue. If the head is presenting and has descended through the inlet, it often can be felt plainly through the fornices. If the placenta covers the entire lower segment, the examiner can palpate nothing but a boggy mass; however, if only a portion of the wall is involved, he may feel the head through one fornix and the soft placenta on the opposite side if the presenting part can be pushed down far enough to reach it. It is difficult to make a definitive diagnosis by this method, particularly if the soft irregular breech or a shoulder presents, and it should be used only if the cervical canal is closed and the finger cannot be inserted through it without forcing it open.

If the cervix is already open, the examining fingers are inserted through it until either placenta or membranes can be felt over the internal os. If the placenta cannot be palpated directly over the cervical opening, the fingertips are swept around the lower segment as high as they can reach. As soon as the physician detects the placental edge and determines the extent of involvement, he should withdraw his fingers. Further manipulation will only separate more placenta and increase bleeding.

Plate 55

Types of placenta previa

A. Low-lying placenta. Much of the placenta is implanted in the upper portion of the uterus, but the lower edge extends down toward the cervix, where the operator may or may not be able to reach it with his examining finger.

B. Incomplete placenta previa. The bulk of the placenta is in the lower segment of the uterus, and the edge extends past the internal os, partially covering the cervical opening. Upon vaginal examination, the soft placental mass can be felt through the vaginal fornix on the left, and the presenting part might be readily palpated on the right. As the fingers are inserted through the open cervix, the membranes and possibly the presenting part can be felt on the right and the placenta on the left.

C. Complete placenta previa. The placenta covers the entire cervical opening, and neither membranes nor presenting part can be palpated unless the fingers are swept far laterally past the edge of the placenta. Such a maneuver serves no useful purpose, however, and may precipitate profuse bleeding. The fingers should be withdrawn as soon as the examiner can ascertain that the opening is completely covered by placenta.

D. Central placenta previa. The entire placenta is implanted in the lower segment, with its central portion rather than an edge overlying the cervix. This cannot be differentiated from complete placenta previa, as illustrated in **C**, by vaginal palpation.

Plate 55

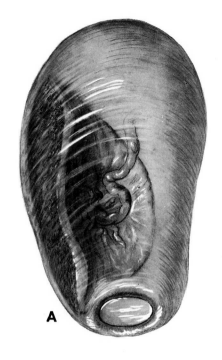

A

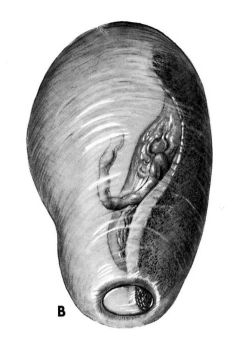

B

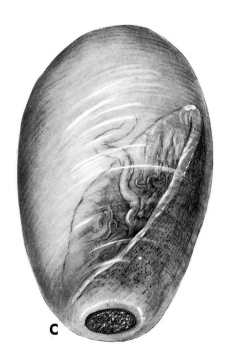

C

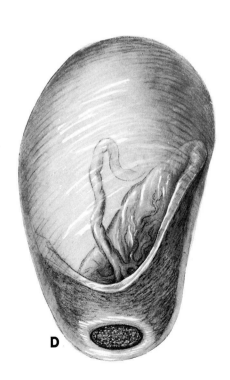

D

Plate 56

Treatment of placenta previa

Complete placenta previa. Almost every patient with complete placenta previa can be most safely delivered by cesarean section. The only possible exception is when total placenta previa is diagnosed during the late second or early third trimester of pregnancy in a patient in labor with the cervix partially dilated and with the infant in a complete breech position. Under such circumstances it is sometimes possible to perforate the placenta and to pull the legs and buttocks through the cervix in order to tamponade and control bleeding. The infant, who has little chance of surviving, almost always dies because the placental circulation is completely disrupted.

If the patient is bleeding profusely when the diagnosis is made, or if the pregnancy is within two or three weeks of term, the operator can proceed with cesarean section at once. If the pregnancy is of less than thirty-six weeks' duration and bleeding is minimal, delivery should be delayed in the interests of the baby. By delaying delivery for even a week or two, a premature infant who might not yet be able to survive outside the uterus may mature and develop enough to live. Sometimes the persistence of bleeding or intermittent hemorrhages will force the operator to empty the uterus rather than to procrastinate further.

Incomplete placenta previa. The time at which a patient with incomplete placenta previa is delivered also is determined by the duration of pregnancy and the amount of bleeding. Many patients, particularly those in whom much of the cervical opening is covered with placenta, and almost all primigravidas are best delivered by cesarean section, but some can be delivered vaginally. Delivery from below may be considered if the cervix is soft, effaced, and partially dilated and the edge of the placenta does not extend much beyond the periphery of the open cervix; if the cervix is closed and uneffaced when it becomes necessary to terminate the pregnancy, abdominal delivery is safer.

A. The bleeding arises from the uterine sinuses beneath the separated area of placenta and from the torn marginal sinus and can be controlled by pressure of the presenting part. If the membranes are intact, it may not be possible for the head to descend enough to tamponade the bleeding vessels. If the membranes are ruptured artificially, the infant's head will usually be pushed down against the placenta and the open sinuses beneath it, and labor will be facilitated.

Plate 56

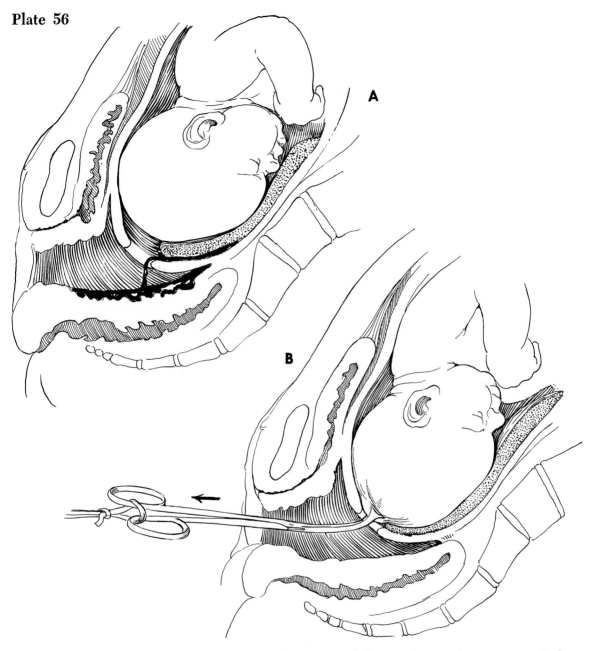

B. Scalp traction. If simple rupture of the membranes does not control the bleeding, further pressure can be applied by pulling the head down against the edge of the placenta. A fold of scalp is grasped with long Allis forceps, a vulsellum clamp, or special Willet forceps, and traction is exerted either manually or with a one- to two-pound weight.

If much of the placenta is compressed by the presenting part, a considerable portion of the fetal circulation is occluded and the infant may die of anoxia. As a consequence, scalp traction is accompanied by a high fetal mortality and should usually be chosen when the infant already is damaged or when the pregnancy is of twenty-eight to thirty weeks' duration and the infant has little chance to survive.

Plate 57

Braxton Hicks version

Braxton Hicks version was used rather extensively in the past to control the bleeding from placenta previa but has now been almost replaced by other methods, particularly cesarean section, which are far less dangerous for both mother and baby. Maternal complications, notably injury, hemorrhage, and infection, occur frequently, and the infant loss is high. Consequently, version should be used rarely and only in carefully selected patients. The procedure is most satisfactory when performed at about the twenty-eighth week of pregnancy, when the baby has almost no chance of surviving and when the main objective is to control the bleeding. The cervix should be dilated at least 4 cm., and the placenta should only partially cover the cervical opening, leaving a free area through which the manipulations can be performed. Deep anesthesia with ether or cyclopropane will eliminate pain and produce uterine relaxation, making the manipulations easier and safer.

A. The head is presenting in an occiput right position and is held well up above the separated placental edge. The cervix is only slightly dilated.

B. The membranes are ruptured artificially, and the index and second fingers are inserted through the opening. After the exact position has been determined, the head is pushed upward well above the brim of the pelvis.

C. The head is pushed farther upward and toward the right with the fingers of the right hand while the buttocks are pushed toward the left by pressure through the abdominal wall with the left hand.

D. The rotation is continued by combined manipulations with the fingers inside the uterus and the hand outside until one of the feet can be grasped between the fingers.

E. The version is completed by pulling the foot into the vagina, but no attempt is made to extract the baby through the incompletely dilated cervix. The thigh and buttocks compress the placenta and the open sinuses and check the bleeding. The infant often dies of anoxia because so much of its placental circulation is occluded.

A one- or two-pound weight can be attached to the foot to maintain pressure, and labor is allowed to continue until the cervix dilates and the infant is expelled.

Plate 57

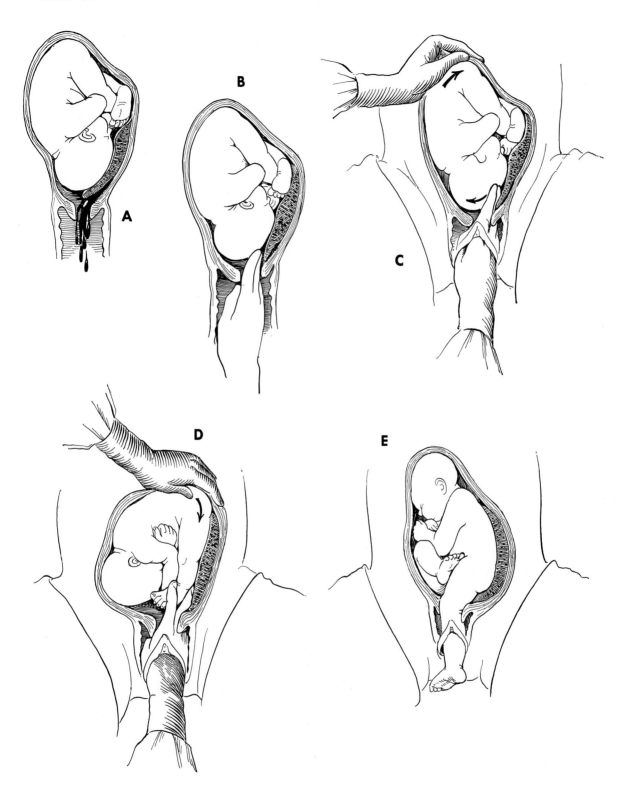

307

Chapter 14

Craniotomy

In past years, before it was possible to perform cesarean section so safely, it often was necessary to perform some sort of destructive operation to reduce the size of the infant enough to permit extraction through the birth canal. At the present time, embryotomy is rarely necessary and cannot often be justified on a living and presumably normal infant. The use of such procedures is limited almost entirely to craniotomy to reduce the size of a hydrocephalic or an aftercoming head, evisceration to empty a distended abdomen or chest, and an occasional cleidotomy to reduce the diameter of the shoulder girdle.

Plate 58

Craniotomy

A. Craniotomy on the aftercoming head. The size of an aftercoming head that is too large to pass through the bony pelvis can be reduced by puncturing the skull and evacuating the contents. Deep anesthesia, either spinal or inhalation, is necessary to relax the voluntary muscles and to eliminate pain.

The infant's body is pulled downward and back by an assistant in an effort to increase the available room anteriorly. After the position of the head has been determined accurately, the blades of the Smellie perforator are introduced into the anterior vagina, and the tip is guided upward to the skull along the fingers of the operator's left hand. Obviously the operator must be careful not to injure the maternal tissues during the introduction of the instrument. The blades are pushed through the lambdoidal suture line or any other readily available opening between the skull bones, and the defect is enlarged by opening and closing the blades in the perforated area. The hydrocephalic head will collapse as the fluid drains through the hole. If the head is of normal size, it will probably be necessary to fragment the brain with the perforator.

Plate 58

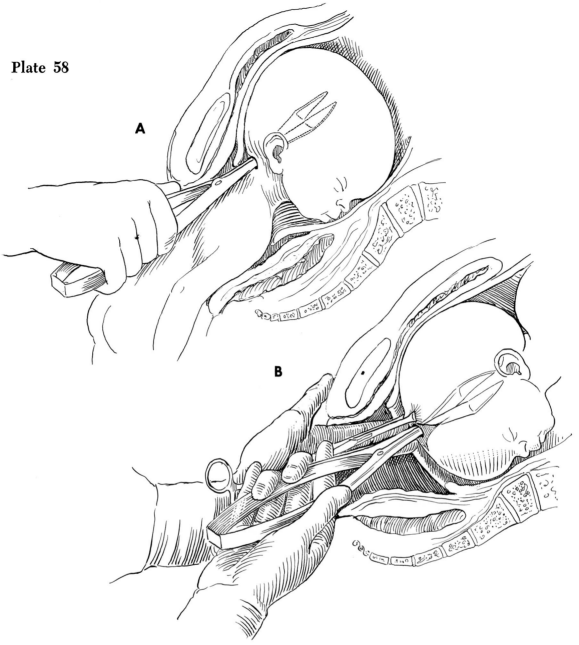

An alternative method for emptying the aftercoming head is to perforate it from beneath the chin. The infant's body is elevated anteriorly over the pubis, and the perforator is introduced through the posterior pelvis and pushed upward into the skull through the submandibular soft tissues.

B. Perforation of the forecoming head. The scalp is grasped with long Allis forceps or a tenaculum with which traction is applied by an assistant to steady it in the inlet. The tip of the Smellie perforator is directed upward with the fingers in the vagina until it is in position against the anterior fontanel or in a suture line. It is pushed into the cavity of the skull by firm pressure, and the opening is enlarged and the brain destroyed with the blades. This reduces the size of the head and permits it to descend through the pelvis. When a fontanel or suture line is not readily available, the blades can be pushed directly through the parietal bone. Sometimes the perforator can be introduced more easily if the skin overlying the selected site is cut with scissors.

The head of the living hydrocephalic infant can be emptied without destroying it, as is almost inevitable when the perforator is used. The scalp is grasped with forceps to steady the head, and a long 15-gauge needle or a small trocar is inserted through the fontanel or a suture line into the distended ventricle. The fluid is drained off or aspirated, permitting the head to collapse and descend. This procedure can be performed through a cervix which is dilated only a few centimeters and offers little risk for the mother.

Index